GERD DIET COOKBOOK FOR BEGINNERS

The Complete Quick and Easy-to-Make Healthy Acid Reflux and Gastric Acid-Friendly Recipes to Beat Heartburn

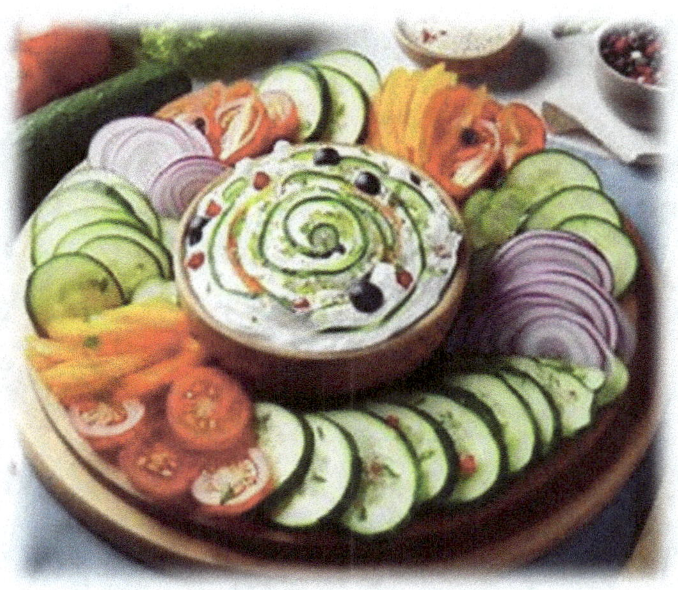

Sharon D. Newsome

Copyright ©2023 Sharon D. Newsome

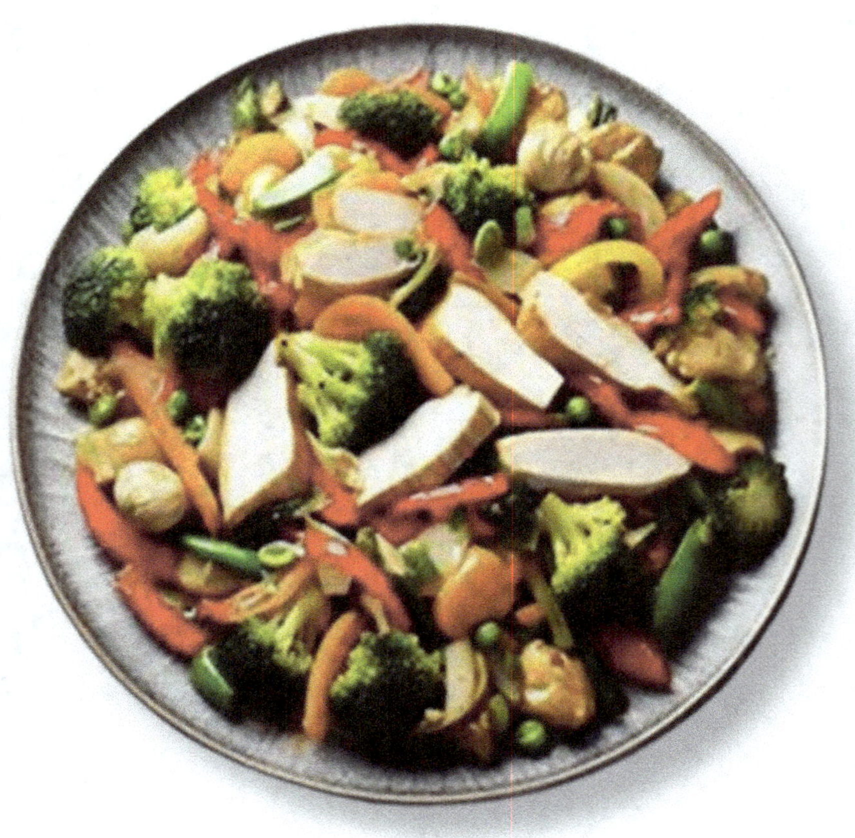

TABLE OF CONTENTS

INTRODUCTION

Imagine going through each day with a throbbing ache, a continual reminder that your body was at battle with itself. This was Debby's everyday life as a vivacious lady in her late thirties trapped in the grasp of Gastroesophageal Reflux Disease (GERD). For years, she endured restless nights, stomach acid regurgitation, and a sense of powerlessness as GERD reduced her quality of life. There appeared to be no way out of the misery and pain that GERD had brought into her life.

But, as if by chance, Debby came across a life-changing remedy - a book that quickly became her GERD sanctuary. The book, was her guiding light during her darkest hours.

Debby's rehabilitation journey started with the first few chapters of the book. She began to have a better understanding of her disease and discovered that dietary modifications may be the key to her treatment. She learned to enjoy meals without fear of penalties thanks to excellent dishes and competent instruction. She no longer had to miss family gatherings or social occasions because of her illness.

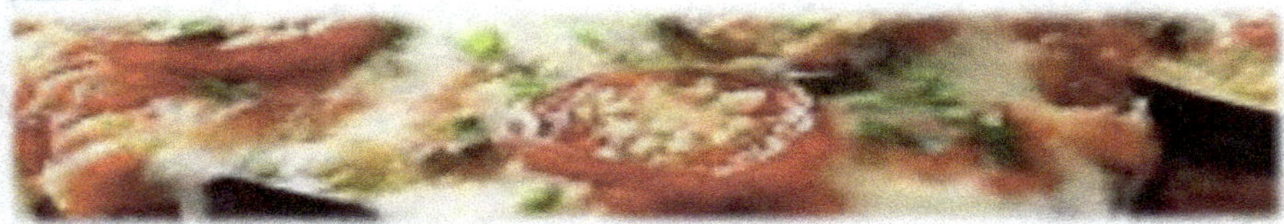

The transformation was astounding. Debby's GERD symptoms progressively reduced as she continued to follow the advice in the book. No more antacids, no more insomnia. She was finally able to recover control of her health, allowing her to live life to the fullest. Debby's newfound wellbeing inspired her to share her accomplishment with others, and soon a ripple effect of relief began to spread.

We shall go on a path of change in this book, not just for Debby, but for all others who have struggled with GERD. We will discover the keys of not just managing but also defeating Gastroesophageal Reflux Disease as we begin on this journey. Debby's story is just one of many that demonstrate the life-changing power of a well-planned GERD diet.

In the following pages, you will also find useful guidance and delightful recipes that have been precisely prepared to bring GERD relief. This book will be your trusty friend as you navigate the treacherous waters of Gastroesophageal Reflux Disease. It's more than a cookbook; it's a lifeline, a road map to greater health, and proof of the power of eating.

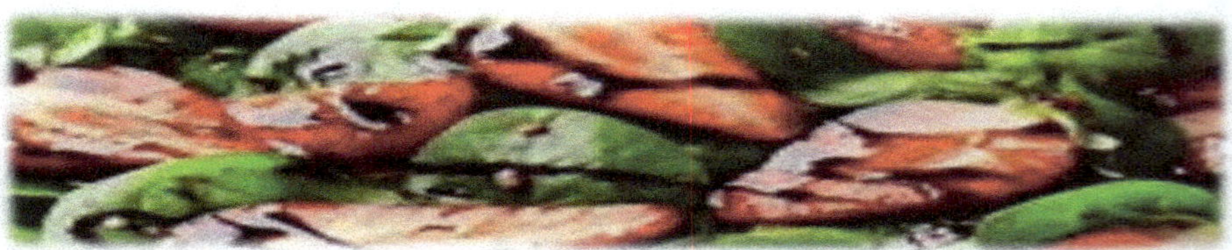

CHAPTER ONE

UNDERSTANDING GERD

What is Gastroesophageal Reflux Disease?

At its core, Gastroesophageal Reflux Disease (GERD) is a complex, often debilitating condition that affects millions worldwide. It's vital to understand the mechanics of GERD to manage it effectively. Simply put, GERD is a chronic disorder where stomach acid flows back into the oesophagus. This backflow occurs due to the weakening of the lower esophageal sphincter (LES), the muscular ring separating the stomach and the esophagus.

Imagine the LES as a guardian gate: when it functions optimally, it prevents the stomach's acidic contents from ascending into the sensitive lining of the esophagus. However, in individuals with GERD, this gate malfunctions, allowing stomach acid to create a burning sensation, often referred to as heartburn.

Common Symptoms and Triggers

The symptoms of GERD are more than just discomfort; they can significantly impact one's quality of life. Heartburn, the hallmark symptom, is characterized by a fiery sensation behind the breastbone. But GERD's reach extends beyond this, manifesting in a range of symptoms such as regurgitation, a sour taste in the mouth, chronic cough, and difficulty swallowing.

Understanding the triggers is essential. Certain foods, Stress, obesity, smoking, and even pregnancy can exacerbate GERD symptoms. As we progress, we'll explore how dietary choices can serve as both triggers and influential allies in managing GERD.

The Impact of Diet on GERD

Diet plays a pivotal role in the course of GERD. The saying, "You are what you eat," couldn't be more accurate. Specific foods and eating habits can either soothe or stoke the flames of GERD. Understanding these dynamics is crucial.

For example, citrus fruits, caffeine, fatty foods, and chocolate are known to relax the LES, facilitating acid reflux. Conversely, a diet rich in whole grains, lean proteins, and fresh produce can contribute to symptom relief. We will dissect the relationship between dietary choices and GERD in subsequent chapters.

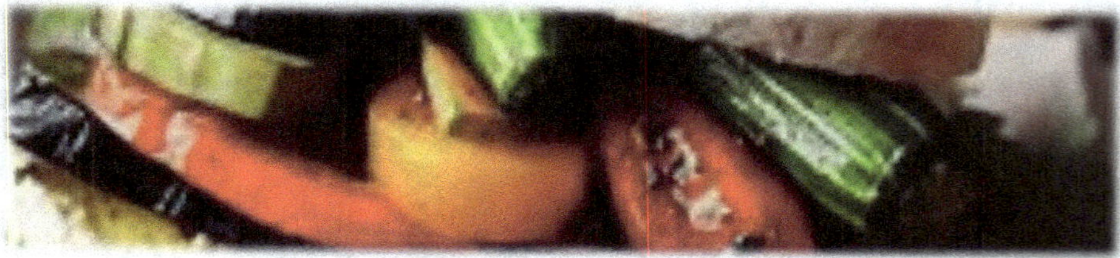

Benefits of a Well-Planned GERD Diet

A well-structured GERD diet offers much more than symptom relief. It can enhance your overall well-being. Imagine experiencing the joy of a meal without fearing the aftermath. A GERD-friendly diet can empower you to reclaim your life, free from the constraints of heartburn and discomfort.

Not only does it alleviate immediate discomfort, but it can also lower the risk of complications, such as esophageal damage and Barrett's esophagus. Additionally, it can lead to better sleep, improved digestion, and even weight management. By following a well-planned GERD diet, you're not just managing symptoms; you're embracing a healthier, more vibrant life.

By gaining a comprehensive understanding of these aspects, you'll be equipped with the knowledge needed to make informed choices and take control of your GERD journey. Your will appreciate the depth of information, enhancing the value and uniqueness of this book.

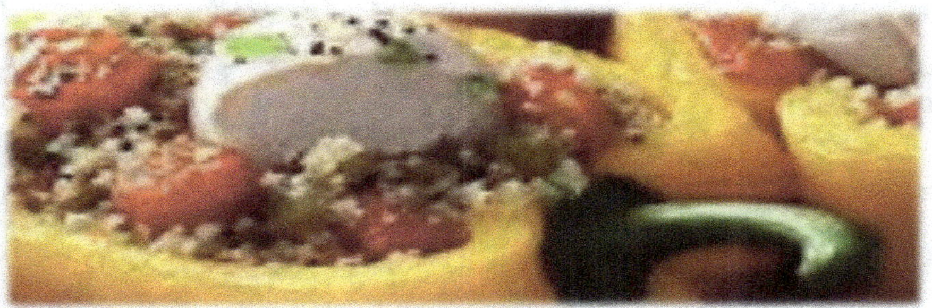

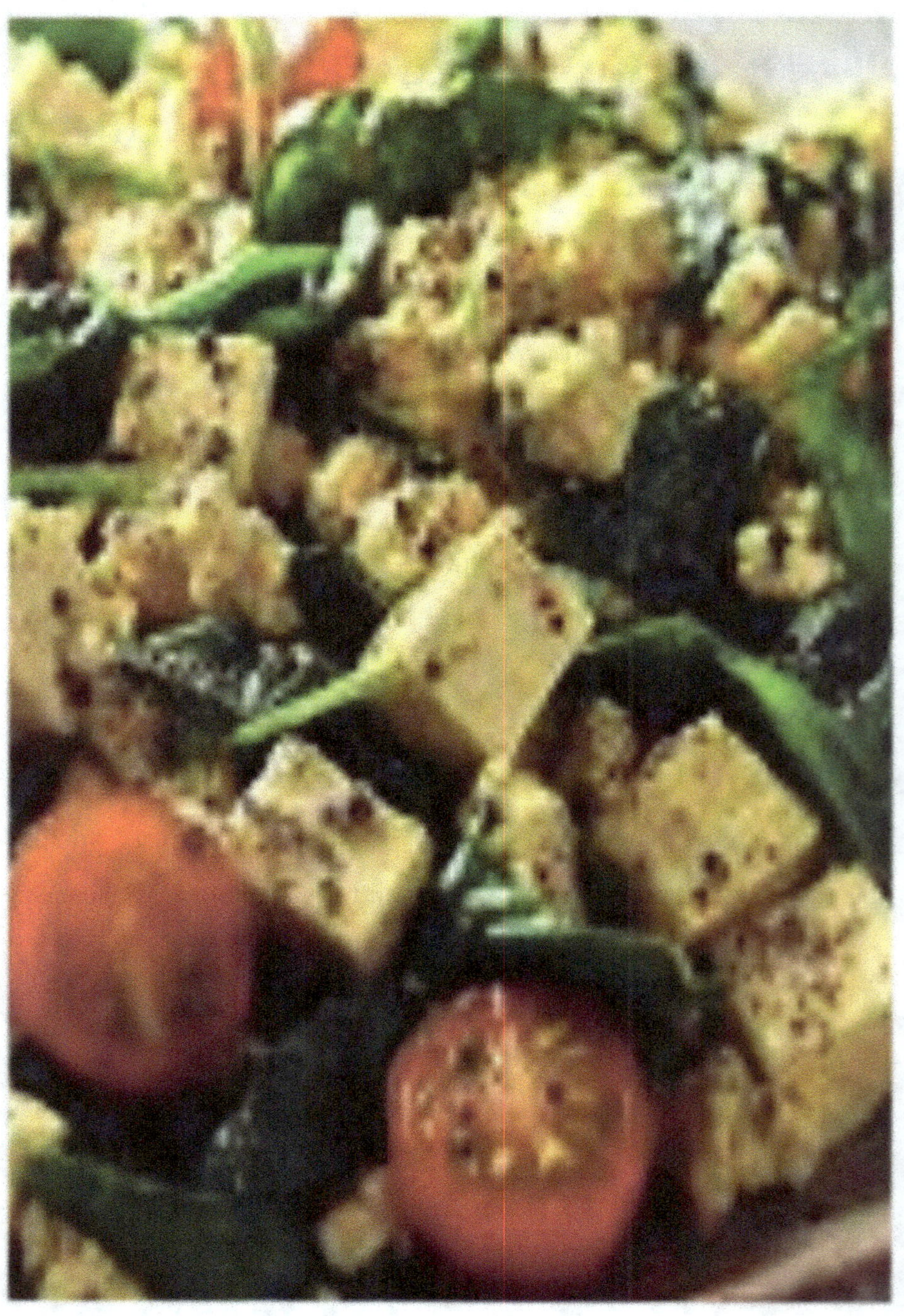

CHAPTER TWO

THE BASICS OF A GERD DIET

General Guidelines and Principles for a Successful GERD Diet Plan

If you suffer from acid reflux or gastroesophageal reflux disease (GERD), you may be wondering what you can do to ease your symptoms and improve your quality of life. One of the most critical factors that can help you manage your condition is your diet. What you eat and how you eat can have a significant impact on how often and how severe your reflux episodes are.

A GERD diet plan is a personalized approach that takes into account your individual needs, preferences, and triggers. However, there are some general guidelines and principles that can help you create a GERD diet plan that works for you. Below are some of them:

1. **Eat Smaller, More Frequent Meals throughout the Day and Drink Plenty of Water.** Eating smaller quantities of food can help prevent overeating and reduce pressure on your stomach, which can trigger reflux. Similarly, water can help dilute the acid in your stomach and flush it out of your system. Aim for at least 8 glasses

of water per day. You can also add some lemon juice or apple cider vinegar to your water to make it more alkaline.

2. Eat Slowly and Mindfully: Take small bites and chew your food well before swallowing. Avoid distractions such as TV or phone while eating. Avoiding distractions can help you enjoy your food more and prevent overeating. It can also help digestion and prevent reflux by diluting the acid in your stomach.

3. Avoid Carbonated Drinks: Carbonated drinks such as soda or sparkling water can cause gas and bloating in your stomach, which can push the acid up into your esophagus.

4. Limit Alcohol Intake: Alcohol can relax the LES and increase the production of acid in your stomach. It can also interfere with your sleep quality and cause dehydration. If you do drink alcohol, limit yourself to one drink per day for women and two drinks per day for men.

5. Avoid Caffeine Intake: Caffeine can stimulate the production of acid in your stomach and keep you awake at night. It can also irritate your esophagus if you have reflux. If you do consume caffeine, limit yourself to one cup of coffee or tea per day and avoid drinking it in the evening.

6. Eat Your Last Meal At Least Three Hours before Bedtime: This can give your stomach enough time to empty and digest your food before you lie down. You can also have a light snack before bed if you feel hungry, such as a banana, a yogurt, or a handful of nuts.

7. Elevate Your Head While Sleeping: This can help gravity keep the acid down in your stomach and prevent it from reaching your esophagus. You can use extra pillows, a wedge, or an adjustable bed to raise your head by 6 to 8 inches.

8. Sleep on Your Left Side: This can help the stomach contents stay away from the LES and reduce the pressure on your stomach. Sleeping on your right side can have the opposite effect and worsen your reflux.

9. Avoid Smoking: Smoking can weaken the lower esophageal sphincter (LES), which is the muscle that prevents the acid from going back up into your esophagus. Smoking can also increase the production of acid in your stomach and cause inflammation in your esophagus.

10. Monitor Your Symptoms and Triggers: Keeping a food diary can help you identify which foods and drinks cause or worsen your reflux, as well as other factors such as Stress, exercise, or medication. You can then avoid or limit these triggers as much as possible.

Foods to Avoid and Foods to Eat for GERD

Some foods and drinks can relax the LES or increase the amount of acid in your stomach, making reflux more likely. These include spicy, fatty, fried, acidic, or caffeinated foods and drinks, such as coffee, chocolate, alcohol, mint, citrus fruits, tomatoes, garlic, onion, etc.

Other foods and drinks that can help strengthen the LES or neutralize the acid in your stomach, making reflux less likely include, high-fiber foods such as whole grains, fruits, vegetables, nuts, and seeds, as well as alkaline foods such as bananas, melons, cauliflower, fennel, and herbal teas.

However, not everyone reacts the same way to different foods and drinks. Some people may be more sensitive or tolerant to certain foods than others. Therefore, it is essential to experiment with different foods and drinks and find out what works best for you. Consider consulting a registered dietitian or nutritionist who can help you create a balanced and varied GERD diet plan that meets your nutritional needs.

Lifestyle Changes and Habits to Support a GERD Diet

Besides following a GERD diet plan, there are some lifestyle changes and habits that can help you manage your condition and improve your overall health and well-being. These include:

1. **Exercise Regularly:** Exercise can help you maintain a healthy weight, which can reduce the pressure on your stomach and prevent reflux. Exercise can also help you relieve Stress, which can trigger reflux. Aim for at least 30 minutes of moderate physical activity per day, such as walking, cycling, swimming, or dancing. However, avoid exercising right after eating or doing exercises that involve bending or lying down, as these can cause reflux.

2. **Manage Stress Effectively:** Stress can affect your digestion and cause your stomach to produce more acid. Stress can also make you more sensitive to pain and discomfort. Therefore, it is essential to find healthy ways to cope with Stress, such as meditation, yoga, breathing exercises, hobbies, or social support.

3. **Lose Weight If Needed:** Being overweight or obese can increase the pressure on your stomach and weaken the LES, making reflux

more likely. Losing weight can help you reduce your symptoms and lower your risk of complications. However, avoid crash diets or fasting, as these can worsen your reflux. Instead, follow a balanced and sustainable GERD diet plan that helps you lose weight gradually and safely.

4. Monitor Your Symptoms and Triggers: Keeping a food diary can help you track your symptoms and triggers and see how your diet affects your reflux. You can also use a symptom tracker app or a journal to record your symptoms and triggers. This can help you identify patterns and trends and make adjustments to your diet and lifestyle accordingly.

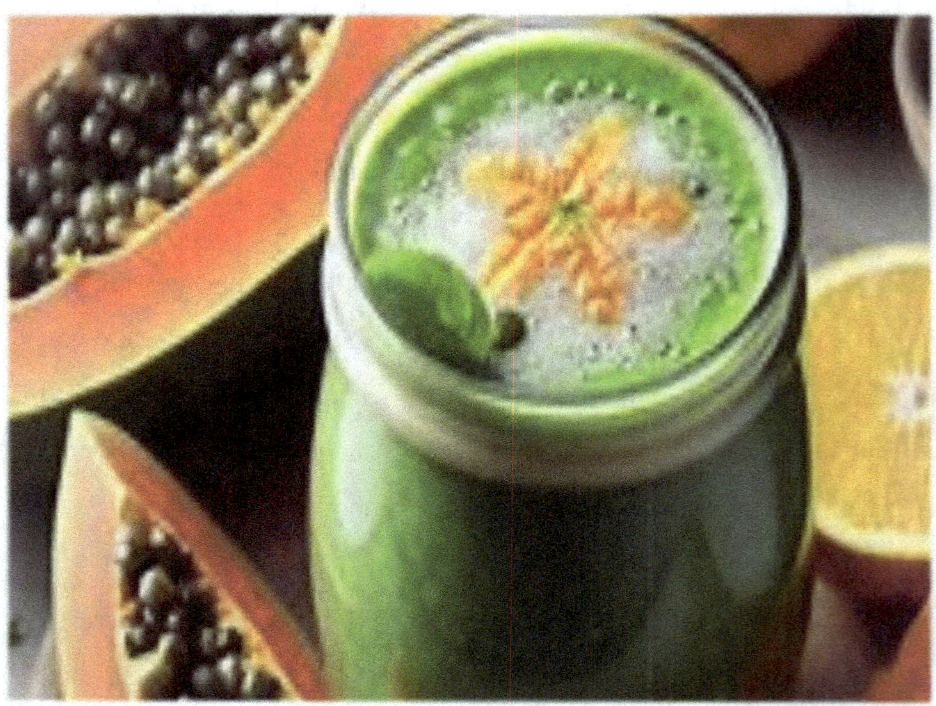

5. Seek Medical Advice If Needed: If your symptoms are severe or persistent, or if you have any signs of complications such as difficulty swallowing, bleeding, weight loss, or anemia, you should see your doctor as soon as possible. Your doctor may prescribe medication or recommend surgery to treat your condition.

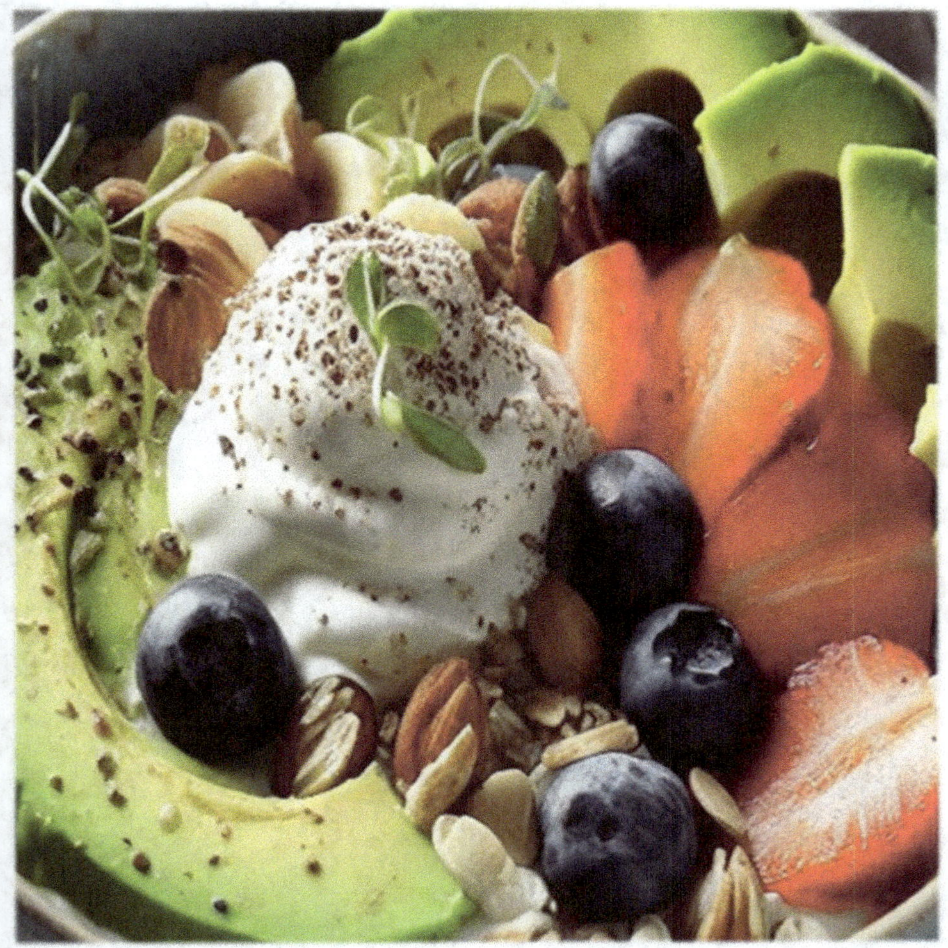

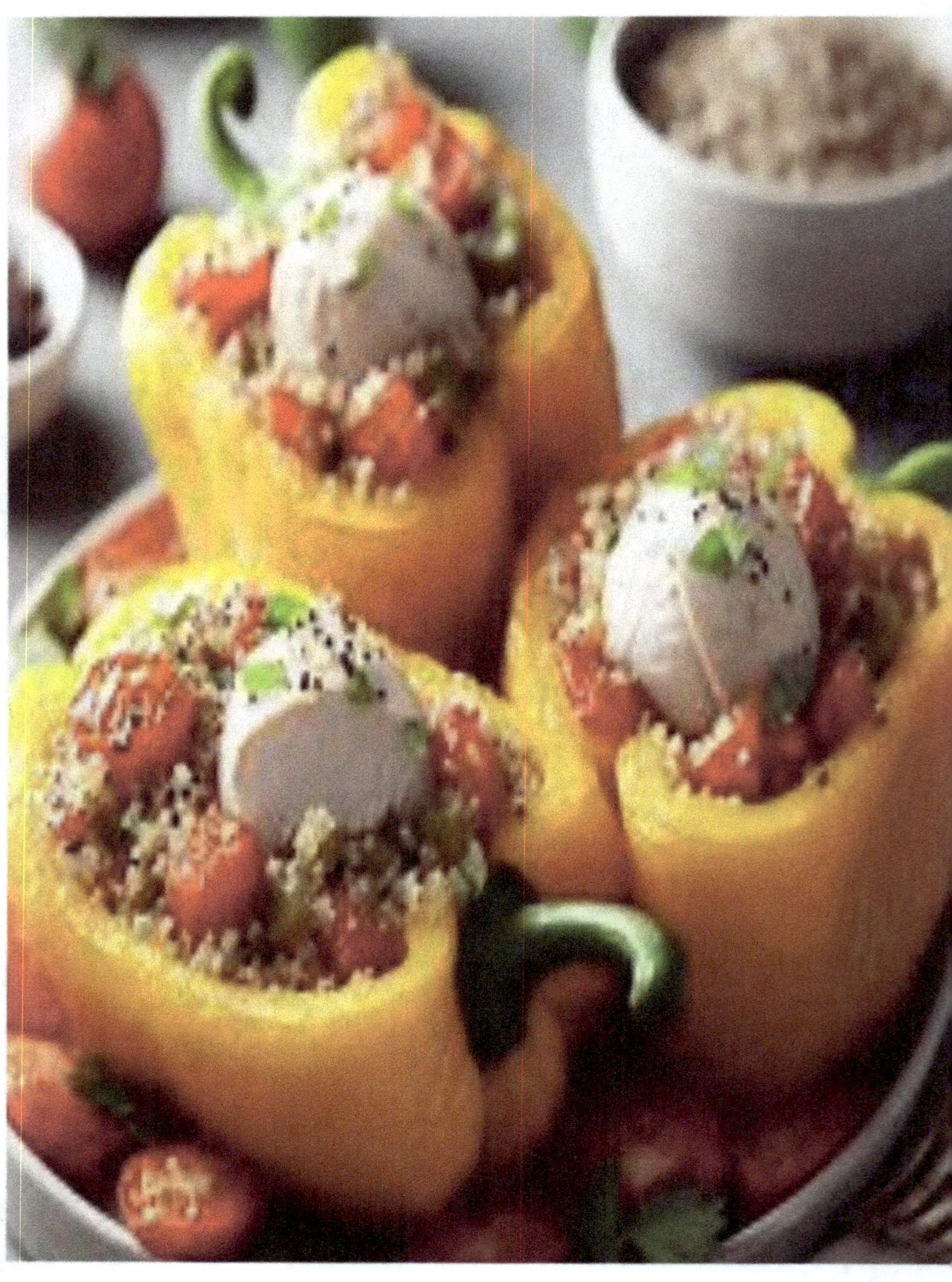

CHAPTER THREE

SETTING THE FOUNDATION

Kitchen Essentials for a GERD Diet

While preparing to do something about your GERD condition, it is essential to have the right tools at your disposal. Invest in a few fundamental kitchen essentials, such as a good set of knives, non-stick cookware, and a food processor.

These items will not only make cooking more manageable but also more enjoyable. Your kitchen can be a powerful ally in your journey to manage GERD. Here are the essentials that will help you create heartburn-free, delicious meals:

1. **Non-Stick Cookware:** Invest in non-stick pans and pots to reduce the need for excessive oil in your cooking. This helps minimize the fat content in your dishes, which can trigger GERD.

2. **Cutting Boards and Utensils:** Designate separate cutting boards and utensils for GERD-friendly foods to avoid cross-contamination. This reduces the risk of introducing acidic residues into your meals.

3. Blender or Food Processor: These appliances are invaluable for creating smooth, easy-to-digest soups and purees from vegetables and fruits.

4. Baking Sheets and Parchment Paper: For healthier baking, opt for baking sheets and parchment paper instead of greasing pans with butter or oil.

Stocking Your Pantry and Fridge

A well-stocked pantry and fridge are your allies in maintaining a GERD diet. Here's what you need:

1. Non-Citrus Fruits: Opt for fruits like bananas, melons, and apples that are less likely to trigger acid reflux.

2. Whole Grains: Keep whole-grain options like brown rice, quinoa, and whole-grain pasta for fiber-rich meals.

3. Lean Proteins: Stock up on lean proteins like skinless poultry, fish, and tofu. These are less likely to cause heartburn.

4. Dairy Alternatives: Opt for non-dairy milk, yogurt, and cheese to reduce fat content. Almond, soy, or oat milk are excellent choices. These are often kinder to the digestive system.

5. Herbs and Spices: Explore the world of herbs and spices that are gentle on your stomach. Ginger, turmeric, and fennel seeds are known for their digestive benefits and can be excellent additions to your GERD-friendly pantry.

6. Vegetables: Load your fridge with non-acidic vegetables such as leafy greens, broccoli, and cauliflower.

7. Water: Stay hydrated with alkaline water, which can help neutralize stomach acid.

8. Fresh Produce: Keep your fridge stocked with fresh fruits and vegetables. Bananas, melons, and leafy greens are excellent choices for GERD sufferers.

9. Healthy Oils: Opt for heart-healthy oils like olive oil or avocado oil. They are not only gentler on your stomach but also provide essential nutrients that support overall health.

10. Herbs and Spices: Stock up on GERD-friendly herbs and spices like oregano, basil, and ginger. These can add flavor without causing heartburn.

Meal Planning for GERD

Effective meal planning is crucial in managing GERD. Here's how to create a GERD-friendly meal plan:

1. Balanced Meals: Aim for balanced meals with a mix of lean protein, whole grains, and plenty of non-acidic fruits and vegetables.

2. Portion Control: Smaller, more frequent meals can prevent overeating, which can trigger heartburn.

3. Dietary Journal: Keep a journal of your meals and any symptoms to identify triggers and patterns.

4. Consistency: Stick to a routine. Regular eating times help regulate digestion and reduce the risk of acid reflux.

Tips for Dining Out with GERD

Dining out doesn't have to be a challenge with GERD. Here are some tips:

1. Choose Wisely: Pick restaurants with GERD-friendly options and avoid spicy, greasy, or citrus-heavy dishes.

2. Ask for Modifications: Don't hesitate to request adjustments to your meal, like no tomato sauce or smaller portion sizes.

3. Share Dishes: Split dishes with a friend or family member to control portion sizes.

4. Avoid Triggers: Steer clear of alcohol, caffeine, and carbonated beverages during your meal.

These foundations for a GERD diet are vital for your journey to better health.

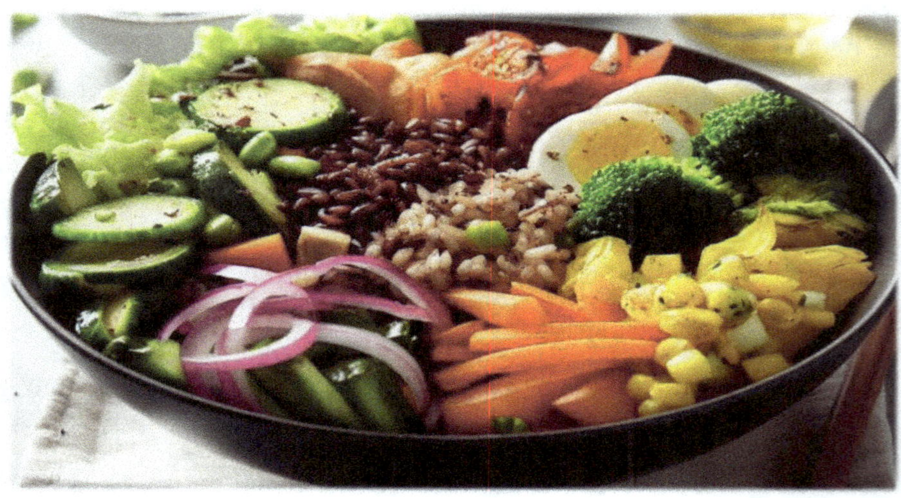

CHAPTER FOUR

28-DAYS MEAL PLAN

This four-week GERD diet meal plan provides a diverse range of meals, and is designed to minimize trigger foods, ensuring that you don't repeat any recipes. Continue to monitor your symptoms to know how your body responds to these meals and make any necessary adjustments based on your body's response. As always, consult with a healthcare professional for personalized dietary recommendations.

Week 1:

Day 1:

- Breakfast: GERD-friendly smoothie (e.g., banana, almond milk, spinach)

- Lunch: Grilled chicken salad with greens and olive oil dressing

- Snack: Sliced melon

- Dinner: Baked salmon with asparagus and quinoa

Day 2:

- Breakfast: Greek yogurt with honey and berries

- Lunch: Turkey and avocado wrap with whole wheat tortilla

- Snack: Almonds

- Dinner: Grilled shrimp with brown rice and steamed broccoli

Day 3:

- Breakfast: Oatmeal with sliced banana

- Lunch: Mixed greens with grilled vegetables and feta cheese

- Snack: Carrot sticks with hummus

- Dinner: Baked cod with roasted sweet potatoes and green beans

Day 4:

- Breakfast: Scrambled eggs with spinach and whole wheat toast

- Lunch: Tuna salad with mixed greens

- Snack: Sliced apples

- Dinner: Stir-fried tofu with brown rice and bok choy

Day 5:

- Breakfast: Cottage cheese with peaches

- Lunch: Quinoa salad with chickpeas and lemon vinaigrette

- Snack: Celery sticks with peanut butter

- Dinner: Roast chicken with mashed potatoes and green peas

Day 6:

- Breakfast: Whole grain cereal with almond milk

- Lunch: Caprese salad with tomato, mozzarella, and basil

- Snack: Sliced papaya

- Dinner: Beef and vegetable stir-fry with brown rice

Day 7:

- Breakfast: Peanut butter and banana on whole wheat toast

- Lunch: Spinach and feta stuffed chicken breast

- Snack: Sliced strawberries

- Dinner: Baked trout with quinoa and asparagus

Week 2:

Day 8:

- Breakfast: Scrambled eggs with diced bell peppers

- Lunch: Turkey and cranberry sauce on whole wheat bread

- Snack: Mixed nuts

- Dinner: Baked tilapia with brown rice and roasted Brussels sprouts

Day 9:

- Breakfast: Whole grain waffles with fresh berries

- Lunch: Caesar salad with grilled chicken

- Snack: Sliced mango

- Dinner: Lentil soup with a side of mixed greens

Day 10:

- Breakfast: Overnight oats with almond butter and sliced peaches

- Lunch: Quinoa and black bean salad with a lime-cilantro dressing

- Snack: Cherry tomatoes with mozzarella

- Dinner: Grilled pork chops with sweet potato wedges and green beans

Day 11:

- Breakfast: Whole grain pancakes with applesauce

- Lunch: Turkey and avocado lettuce wraps

- Snack: Sliced pears

- Dinner: Baked cod with quinoa and sautéed spinach

Day 12:

- Breakfast: Greek yogurt parfait with honey and granola

- Lunch: Mixed greens with grilled shrimp

- Snack: Sliced kiwi

- Dinner: Roast beef with mashed cauliflower and steamed carrots

Day 13:

- Breakfast: Scrambled eggs with diced tomatoes

- Lunch: Spinach and strawberry salad with grilled chicken

- Snack: Mixed berries

- Dinner: Stir-fried tofu with brown rice and broccoli

Day 14:

- Breakfast: Oatmeal with cinnamon and sliced apples

- Lunch: Caprese salad with grilled chicken

- Snack: Sliced peaches

- Dinner: Baked chicken with quinoa and roasted asparagus

Week 3:

Day 15:

- Breakfast: Smoothie with spinach, pineapple, and Greek yogurt

- Lunch: Quinoa and vegetable stir-fry

- Snack: Sliced watermelon

- Dinner: Baked salmon with dill sauce, brown rice, and steamed asparagus

Day 16:

- Breakfast: Oatmeal with sliced strawberries and a drizzle of honey

- Lunch: Grilled chicken Caesar wrap with romaine lettuce

- Snack: Mixed nuts

- Dinner: Turkey meatloaf with mashed sweet potatoes and green beans

Day 17:

- Breakfast: Scrambled eggs with diced bell peppers and a side of salsa

- Lunch: Tuna and white bean salad with lemon-tahini dressing

- Snack: Sliced apricots

- Dinner: Grilled swordfish with quinoa and sautéed kale

Day 18:

- Breakfast: Whole grain waffles with fresh raspberries and Greek yogurt

- Lunch: Spinach and pear salad with walnuts and a balsamic vinaigrette

- Snack: Sliced oranges

- Dinner: Pork tenderloin with roasted butternut squash and broccoli

Day 19:

- Breakfast: Greek yogurt parfait with granola and mango

- Lunch: Quinoa and roasted vegetable salad with hummus dressing

- Snack: Mixed berries

- Dinner: Baked tilapia with couscous and lemon-dill green beans

Day 20:

- Breakfast: Scrambled eggs with sautéed mushrooms

- Lunch: Turkey and cranberry lettuce wraps with avocado

- Snack: Sliced plums

- Dinner: Chicken stir-fry with brown rice and sugar snap peas

Day 21:

- Breakfast: Oatmeal with sliced bananas and almond butter

- Lunch: Mixed greens with grilled shrimp and citrus vinaigrette

- Snack: Sliced cantaloupe

- Dinner: Beef and vegetable kebabs with quinoa and grilled zucchini

Week 4:

Day 22:

- Breakfast: Whole grain pancakes with blueberries and honey

- Lunch: Caprese salad with grilled chicken breast

- Snack: Mixed nuts

- Dinner: Baked cod with lemon-herb quinoa and roasted brussels sprouts

Day 23:

- Breakfast: Smoothie with kale, mango, and chia seeds

- Lunch: Quinoa and black bean salad with lime-cilantro dressing

- Snack: Sliced kiwi

- Dinner: Pork chops with mashed cauliflower and steamed carrots

Day 24:

- Breakfast: Scrambled eggs with diced tomatoes and feta cheese

- Lunch: Spinach and strawberry salad with grilled shrimp

- Snack: Sliced peaches

- Dinner: Baked chicken with brown rice and sautéed spinach

Day 25:

- Breakfast: Whole grain cereal with almond milk and sliced pears

- Lunch: Turkey and avocado lettuce wraps with salsa

- Snack: Sliced cherries

- Dinner: Tofu stir-fry with quinoa and snow peas

Day 26:

- Breakfast: Oatmeal with cinnamon and sliced apples

- Lunch: Mixed greens with grilled swordfish and citrus dressing

- Snack: Sliced grapes

- Dinner: Beef and broccoli stir-fry with brown rice

Day 27:

- Breakfast: Scrambled eggs with diced bell peppers and a side of guacamole

- Lunch: Turkey and cranberry sauce wrap with mixed greens

- Snack: Mixed berries

- Dinner: Baked trout with couscous and lemon-dill green beans

Day 28:

- Breakfast: Greek yogurt with honey and pineapple

- Lunch: Quinoa and vegetable stir-fry with teriyaki sauce

- Snack: Sliced apricots

- Dinner: Roast pork loin with mashed sweet potatoes and asparagus

GERD DIET SHOPPING LIST

Fruits and Vegetables:

- Bananas

- Apples

- Pears

- Melons

- Berries (strawberries, blueberries)

- Papaya

- Avocado

- Spinach

- Kale

- Cucumbers

- Carrots

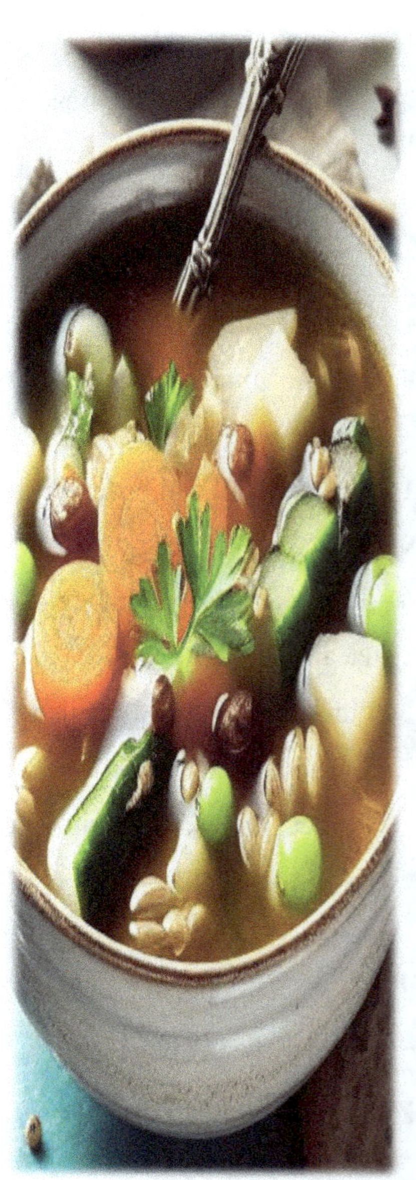

- Broccoli

- Asparagus

- Brussels sprouts

- Zucchini

- Sweet potatoes

- Butternut squash

- Bell peppers

- Green beans

Protein:

- Skinless poultry (chicken, turkey)

- Lean cuts of beef

- Pork loin

- Fish (salmon, cod, mahi-mahi)

- Shrimp

- Tofu

- Eggs

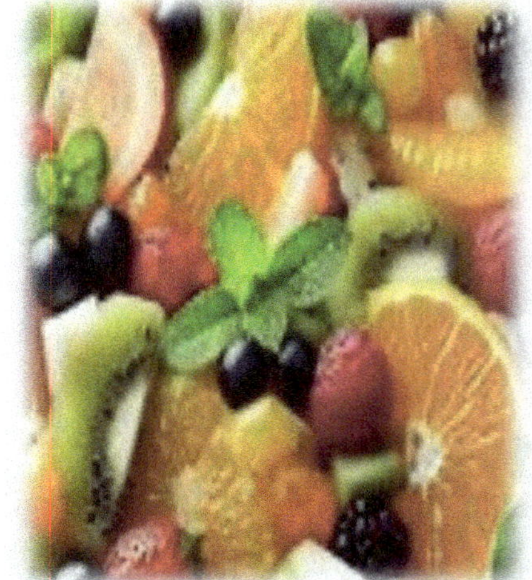

Grains and Bread:

- Oatmeal

- Whole-grain bread (look for low-fat, whole-grain options)

- Quinoa

- Brown rice

- Whole-grain pasta

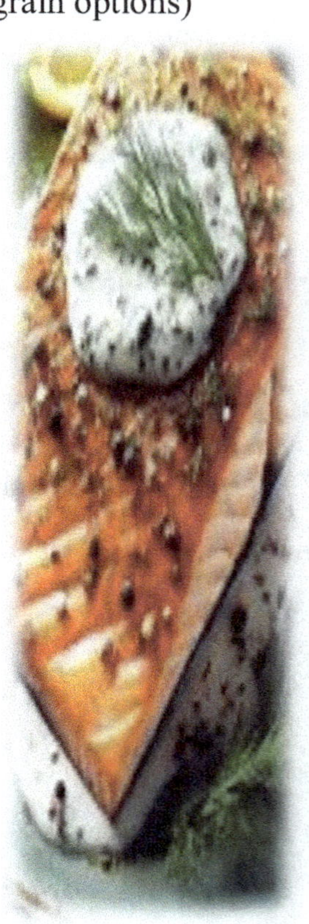

Dairy and Dairy Alternatives:

- Low-fat or non-fat Greek yogurt

- Almond milk (plain, unsweetened)

- Low-fat or non-fat cheese

Legumes:

- Black beans

- Garbanzo beans (chickpeas)

- Lentils

Nuts and Seeds:

- Almonds

- Walnuts

- Chia seeds

Condiments and Sauces:

- Olive oil

- Balsamic vinegar

- Honey

- Dijon mustard

- Low-fat mayonnaise

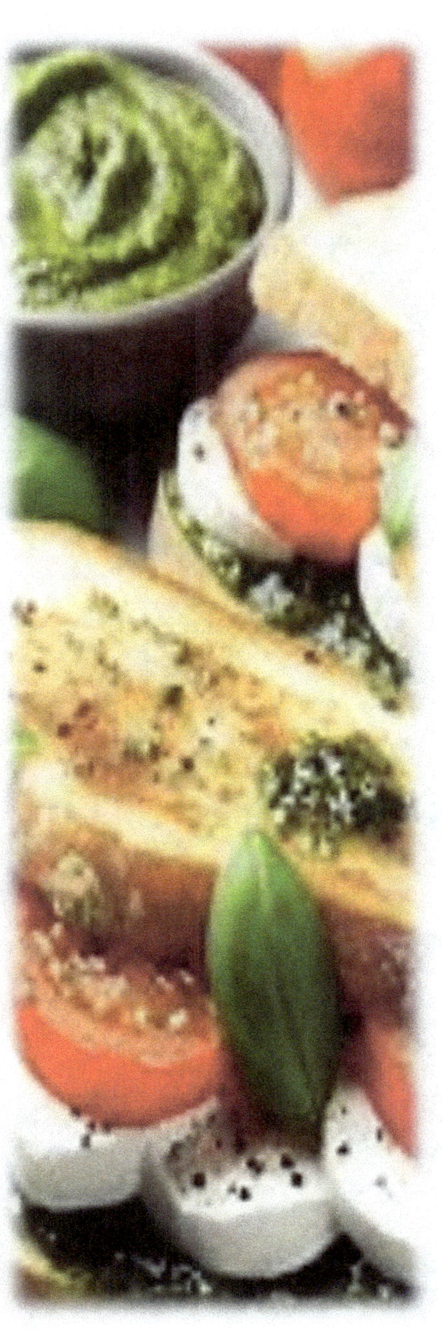

- Tomato sauce (low-acid options)

- Fresh herbs and spices (oregano, basil, thyme, ginger, turmeric)

Beverages:

- Water

- Herbal teas (chamomile, ginger, licorice root)

- Low-acid coffee (if tolerated)

- Aloe vera juice (pure, no added sugar)

Snacks:

- Rice cakes

- Hummus

- Popcorn (plain, air-popped)

- Whole-grain crackers (look for low-fat options)

Sweeteners:

- Stevia

- Maple syrup (in moderation)

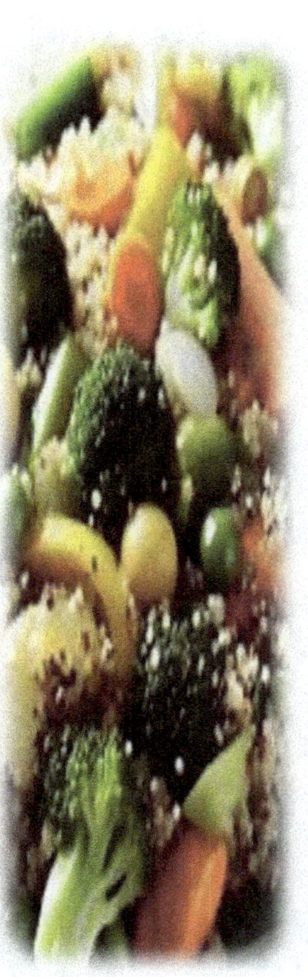

Miscellaneous:

- Low-sodium chicken or vegetable broth

- Low-fat salad dressings

- Apple cider vinegar (use sparingly, if tolerated)

- Low-sodium soy sauce

Always remember to read labels carefully and opt for low-fat, low-acid, and non-spicy options whenever possible. It's essential to choose fresh, whole, and unprocessed foods to minimize the risk of GERD symptoms. Also, consider any personal dietary preferences or restrictions while shopping.

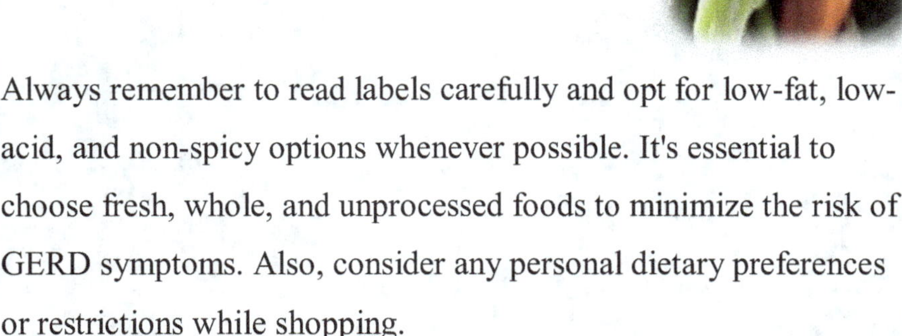

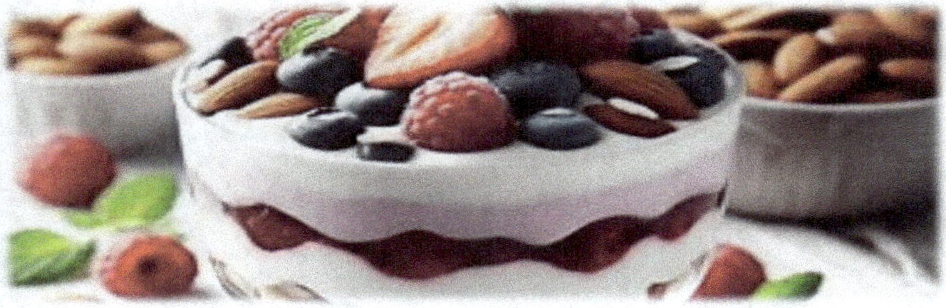

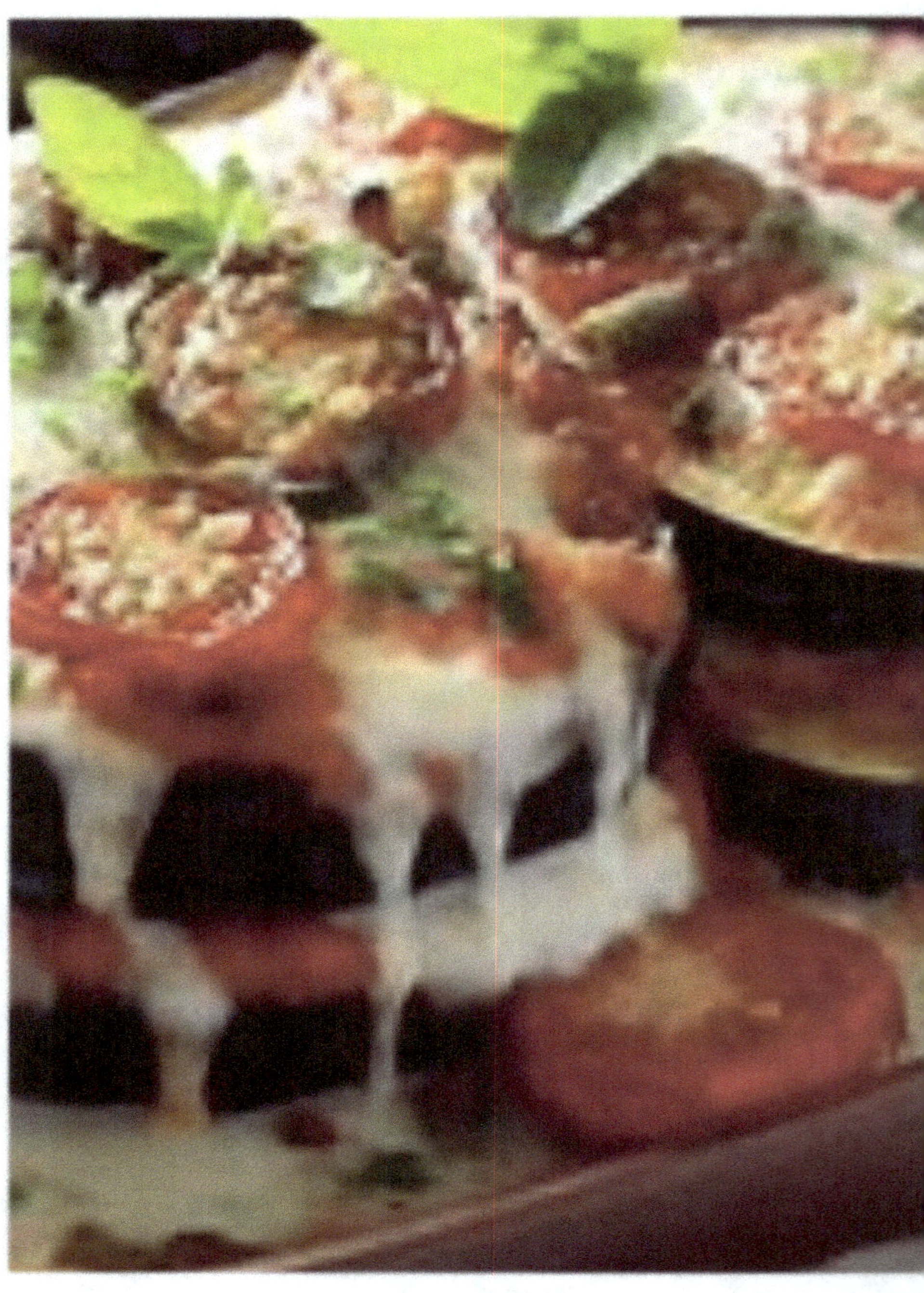

CHAPTER FIVE

GERD FRIENDLY BREAKFAST RECIPES

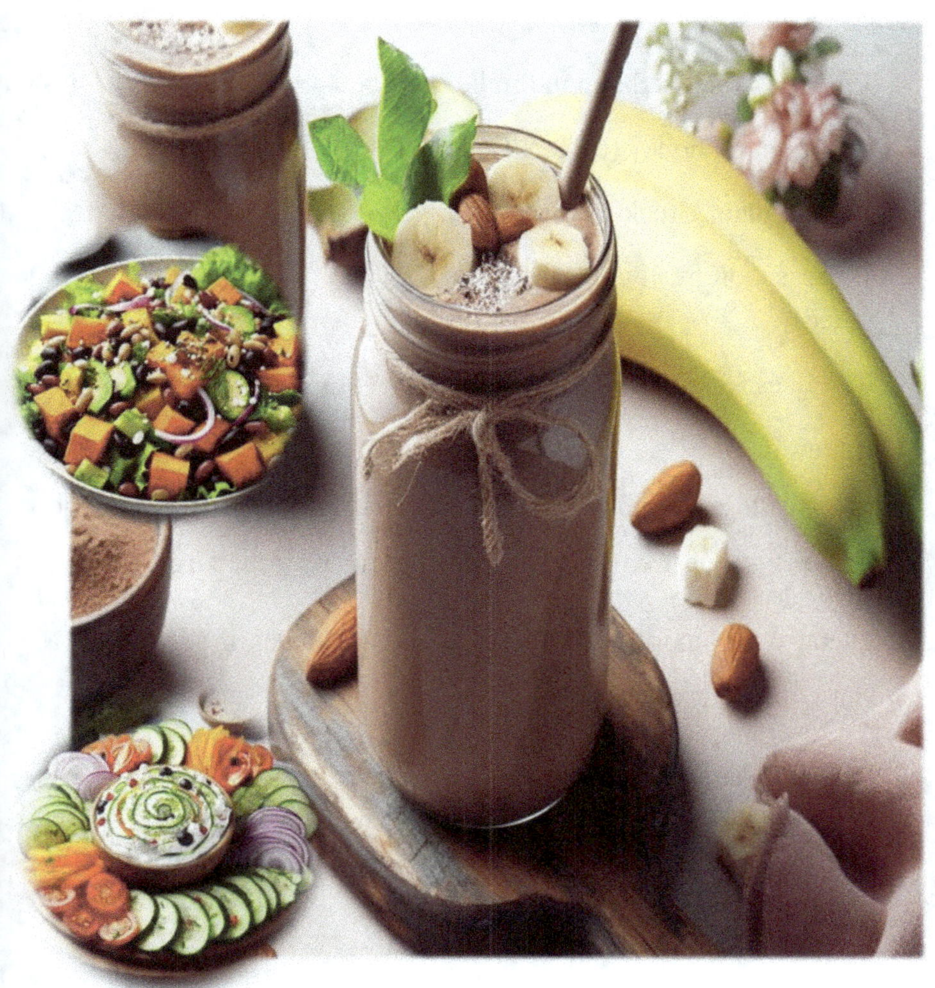

Banana-Berry Breakfast Smoothie

Prep Time: 5 minutes | Servings: 1 | Calories: 220

Ingredients:

- 1 ripe banana

- 1/2 cup mixed berries (blueberries, strawberries, or raspberries)

- 1 cup unsweetened almond milk

- 1 tablespoon honey (optional)

- 1/2 cup plain Greek yogurt

- 1/2 teaspoon fresh ginger (grated)

- Ice cubes (optional)

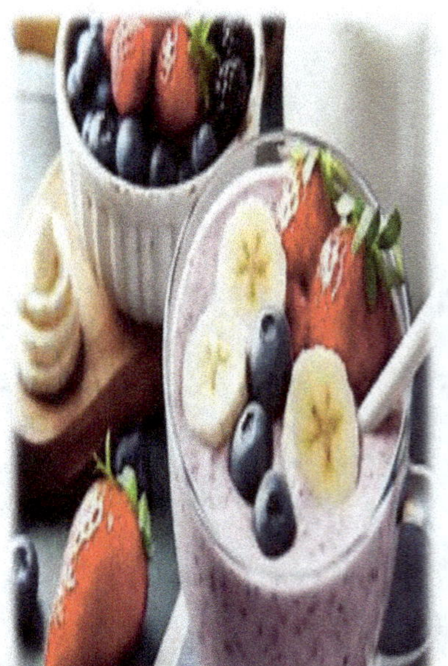

Instruction

1. In a blender, combine the ripe banana, mixed berries, almond milk, honey (if desired), plain Greek yogurt, and grated fresh ginger.

2. Blend until smooth and creamy. Add ice cubes if you prefer a colder consistency.

3. Pour into a glass

4. Enjoy the soothing goodness of this banana-berry breakfast smoothie.

Avocado Toast with Poached Egg

Prep Time: 10 mins | Cook Time: 10 mins | Servings:1 | Cal: 310

Ingredients:

- 1 ripe avocado

- 1 slice whole-grain bread

- 1 large egg

- Salt and pepper to taste

- Fresh herbs (e.g., cilantro or parsley) for garnish

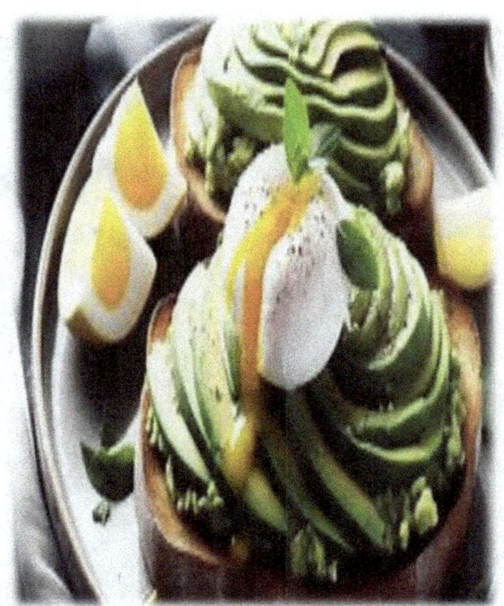

Instructions:

1. Toast the whole-grain bread to your preferred level of crispness.

2. Fill a saucepan with water and bring it to a simmer. Gently slide the egg into the simmering water. Poach for about 3 minutes for a runny yolk.

3. Mash the ripe avocado and spread it on the toasted bread. Season with salt and pepper.

4. Place the poached egg on top of the avocado toast, garnish with fresh herbs, and serve.

Blueberry-Oatmeal Smoothie Bowl

Prep Time: 10 │minutes Servings: 1│ - Calories: 370

Ingredients:

- 1/2 cup old-fashioned oats

- 1/2 cup frozen blueberries

- 1/2 cup plain Greek yogurt

- 1 tablespoon honey

- 1/4 cup unsweetened almond milk

- 1 tablespoon sliced almonds

- Fresh blueberries and a drizzle of honey for garnish

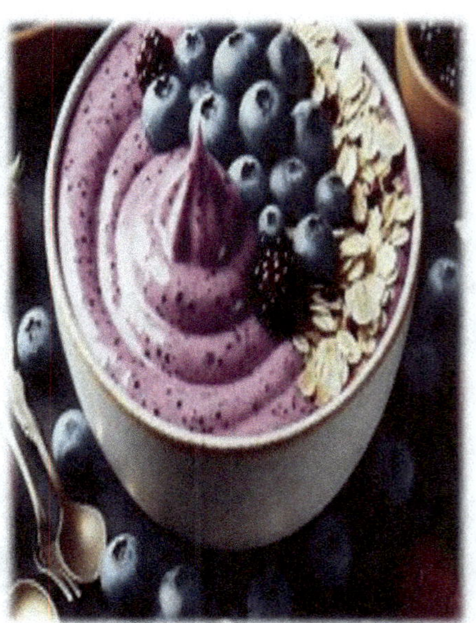

Instructions:

1. In a blender, combine the old-fashioned oats, frozen blueberries, plain Greek yogurt, honey, and unsweetened almond milk.

2. Blend until the mixture is smooth and creamy.

3. Pour the smoothie into a bowl and top with sliced almonds, fresh blueberries, and a drizzle of honey and enjoy.

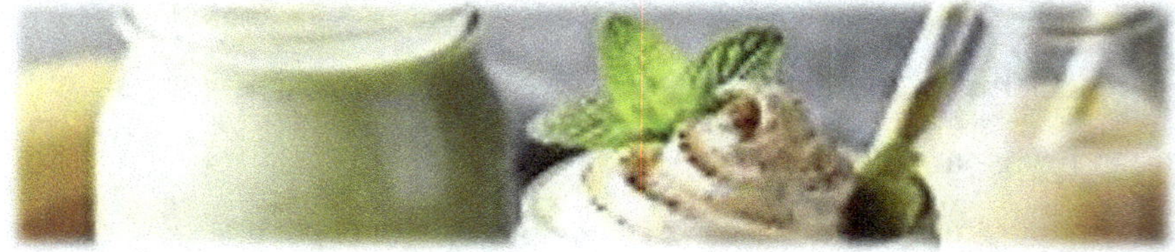

Greek Yogurt Parfait

Prep Time: 5 minutes | Servings: 1 | - Calories: 390

Ingredients:

- 1 cup plain Greek yogurt

- 2 tablespoons honey

- 1/2 cup mixed berries (e.g., strawberries, blueberries, raspberries)

- 1/4 cup granola

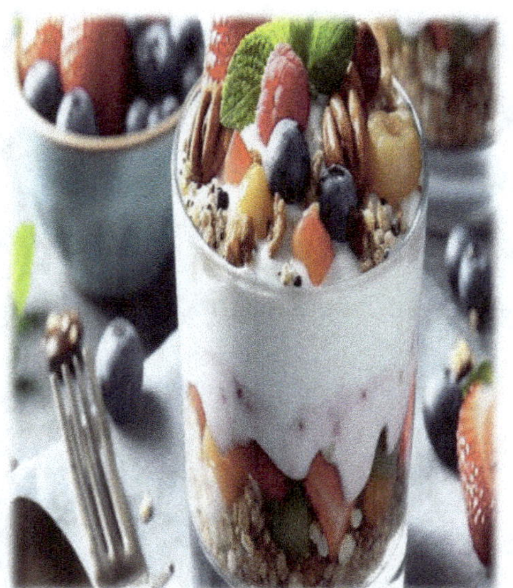

Instructions:

1. In a glass or bowl, begin with a layer of plain Greek yogurt.

2. Drizzle a tablespoon of honey over the yogurt.

3. Add a layer of mixed berries.

4. Sprinkle a portion of granola on top.

5. Repeat the layers until the glass is filled.

6. Finish with a drizzle of the remaining honey.

7. Grab a spoon and enjoy your delicio us Greek yogurt parfait.

Peanut Butter and Banana Overnight

Prep Time: 10 mins (overnight chilling) | Servings: 1 | Cal: 360

Ingredients:

- 1/2 cup old-fashioned oats

- 1 cup unsweetened almond milk

- 1 tablespoon natural peanut butter

- 1 ripe banana, sliced

- 1/2 teaspoon honey

- Chopped peanuts for garnish

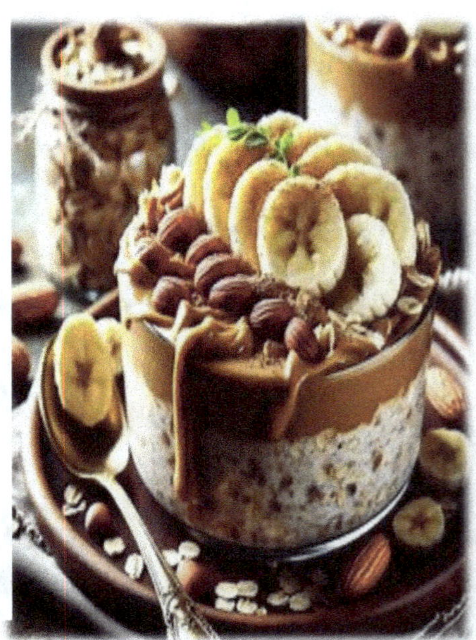

Instructions:

1. In a Mason jar or airtight container, combine the old-fashioned oats and unsweetened almond milk.

2. Stir in the natural peanut butter and sliced banana.

3. Drizzle with honey.

4. Close the container and refrigerate overnight.

5. In the morning, give it a good stir, top with chopped peanuts, and enjoy your peanut butter and banana overnight oats.

Scrambled Tofu with Spinach and Tomatoes

Prep Time: 10 mins | Cook Time: 10 mins | Servings:1 | Cal: 220

Ingredients:

- 1/2 block of firm tofu, crumbled

- 1 cup fresh spinach

- 1 small tomato, diced

- 1/4 teaspoon turmeric

- 1/4 teaspoon paprika

- Salt and pepper to taste

- Fresh parsley for garnish

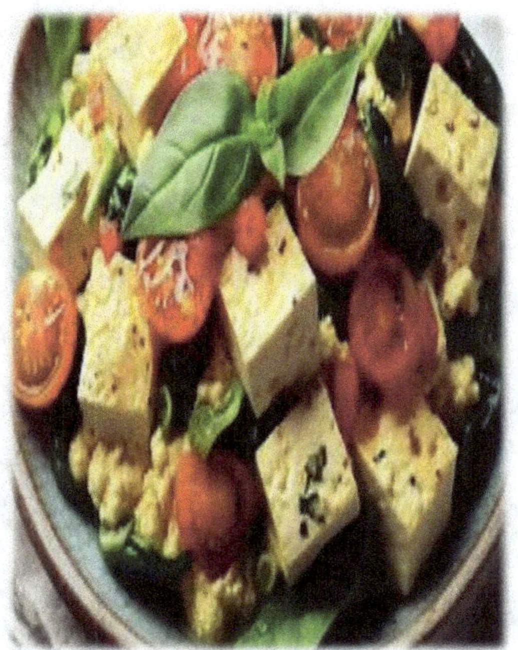

Instructions:

1. In a non-stick skillet, sauté crumbled tofu until slightly browned.

2. Add diced tomatoes and fresh spinach to the skillet and cook until the spinach wilts.

3. Season with turmeric, paprika, salt, and pepper.

4. Garnish with fresh parsley and enjoy your light yet flavorful tofu scramble.

Quinoa Breakfast Bowl

Prep Time: 15 mins | Cook Time: 15 mins | Servings: 1 | Cal: 310

Ingredients:

- 1/2 cup cooked quinoa

- 1/2 cup mixed fresh fruit (e.g., sliced banana, berries, kiwi)

- 1 tablespoon honey

- 1 tablespoon chopped nuts (e.g., almonds, walnuts)

- 1/4 teaspoon cinnamon

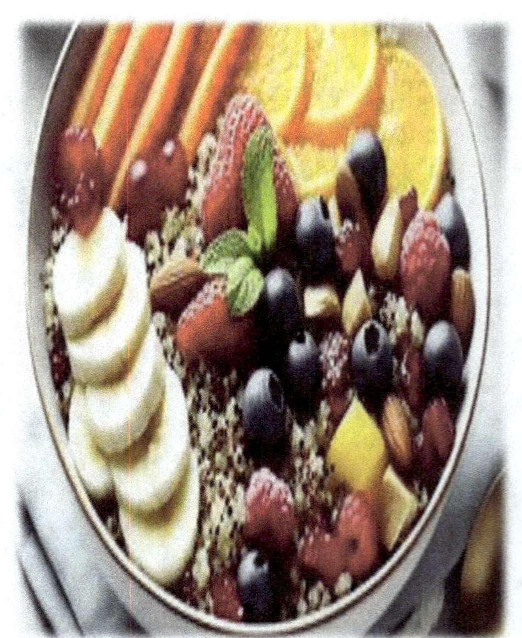

Instructions:

1. In a bowl, combine the cooked quinoa and fresh fruit.

2. Drizzle with honey and sprinkle with chopped nuts.

3. Dust with cinnamon and savor this delightful quinoa breakfast

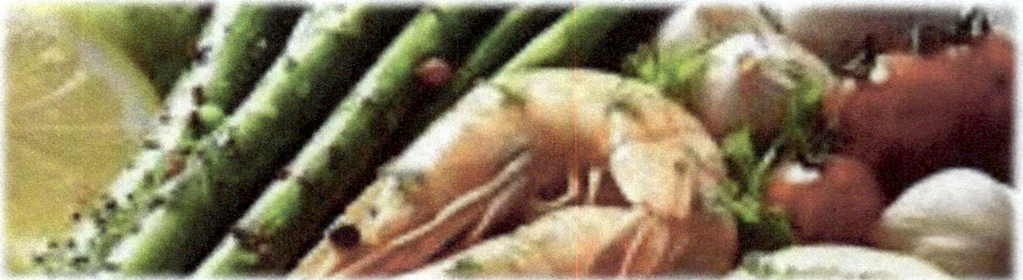

Sweet Potato Hash

Prep Time: 15 mins | Cook Time: 20 mins | Servings: 1 | Cal: 280

Ingredients:

- 1 small sweet potato, diced
- 1/4 red bell pepper, diced
- 1/4 yellow bell pepper, diced
- 1/4 onion, diced
- 1/2 teaspoon paprika
- Salt and pepper to taste
- 1 tablespoon olive oil

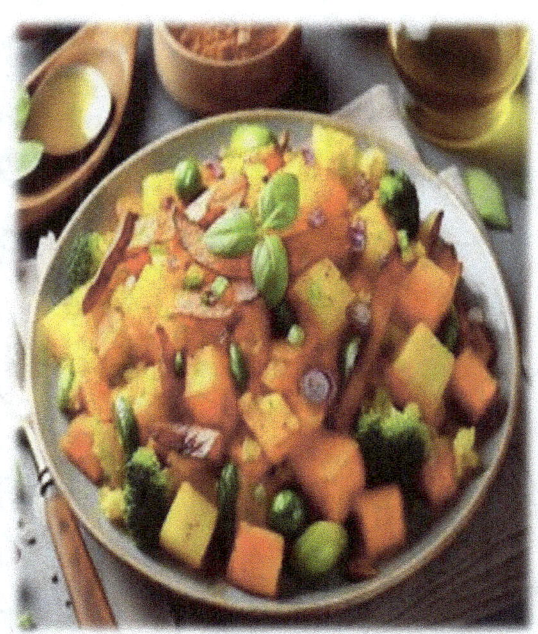

Instructions:

1. Heat olive oil in a skillet and add diced sweet potatoes.

2. Sauté until they start to brown.

3. Add bell peppers and onions, and cook until tender.

4. Season with paprika, salt, and pepper. Serve hot and enjoy.

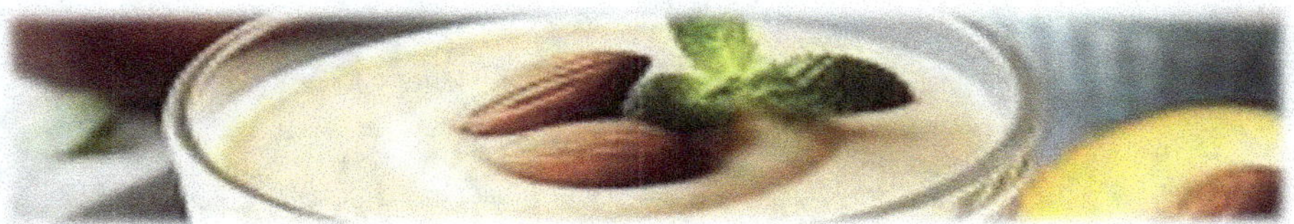

Chia Pudding with Fresh Berries

Prep Time: 5 mins (plus chilling time) │ Servings: 1 │ Cal: 260

Ingredients:

- 3 tablespoons chia seeds

- 1 cup unsweetened almond milk

- 1/2 cup mixed fresh berries (e.g., blueberries, raspberries)

- 1 tablespoon honey

- 1/4 teaspoon vanilla extract

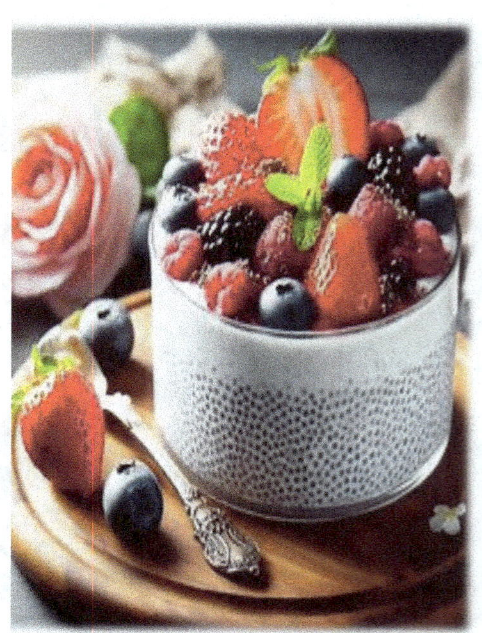

Instructions:

1. In a jar, combine chia seeds and unsweetened almond milk.

2. Add honey and vanilla extract, and stir well.

3. Refrigerate for at least 2 hours or overnight until it thickens.

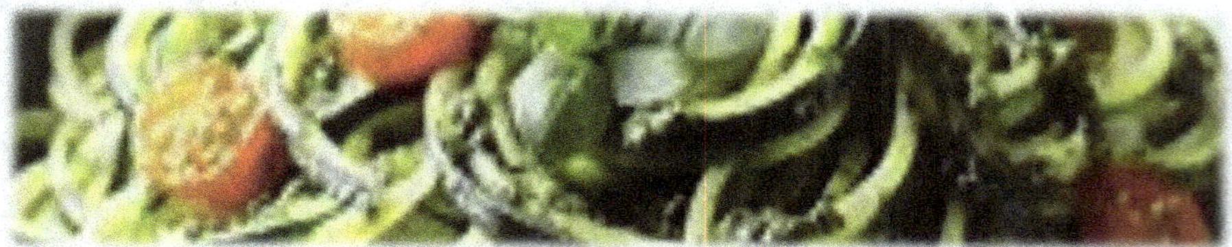

Spinach and Mushroom Omelette

Prep Time: 10 mins | Cook Time: 10 mins | Servings: 1 | Cal: 250

Ingredients:

- 2 large eggs

- 1/2 cup fresh spinach, chopped

- 1/4 cup mushrooms, sliced

- 1/4 onion, chopped, salt and pepper to taste

- 1 teaspoon olive oil

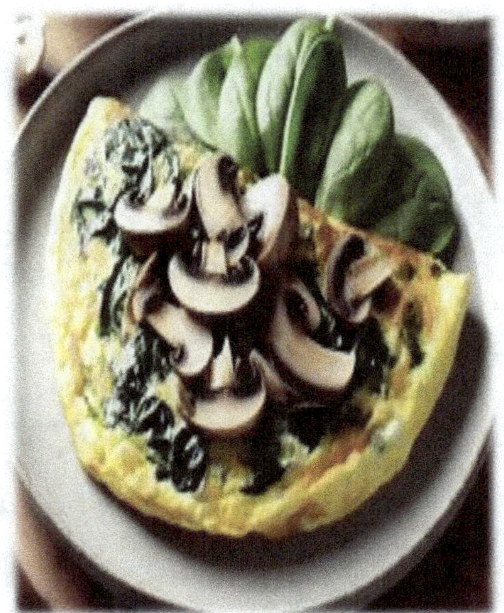

Instructions:

1. Heat olive oil in a skillet. Add onions, mushrooms, and sauté until they're tender.

3. Add chopped spinach and cook until wilted.

4. In a separate bowl, whisk eggs and season with salt and pepper.

5. Pour the egg mixture into the skillet with sautéed veggies.

6. Cook until the omelette is set and golden on both sides. Serve hot.

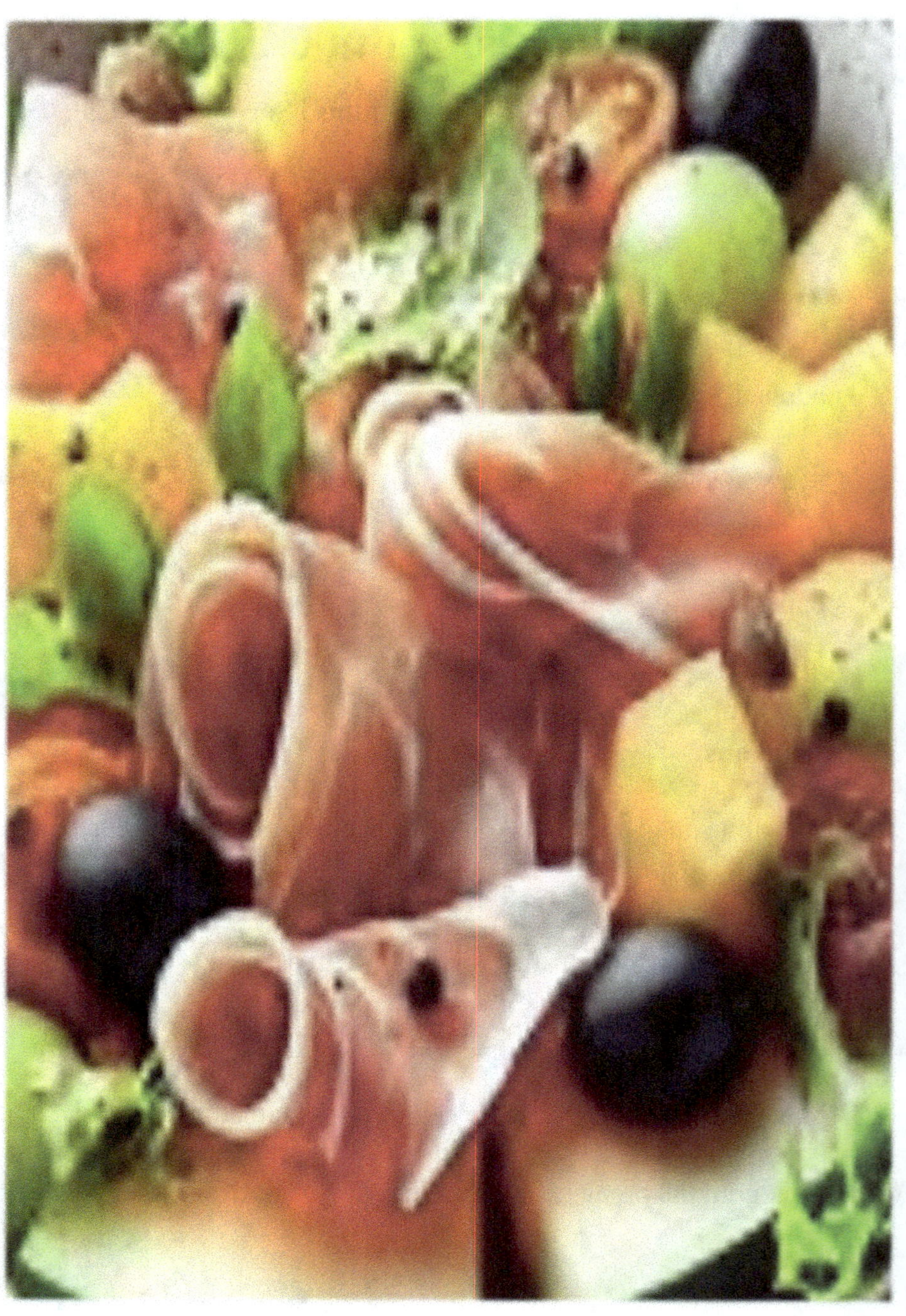

ENERGIZING LUNCH RECIPES

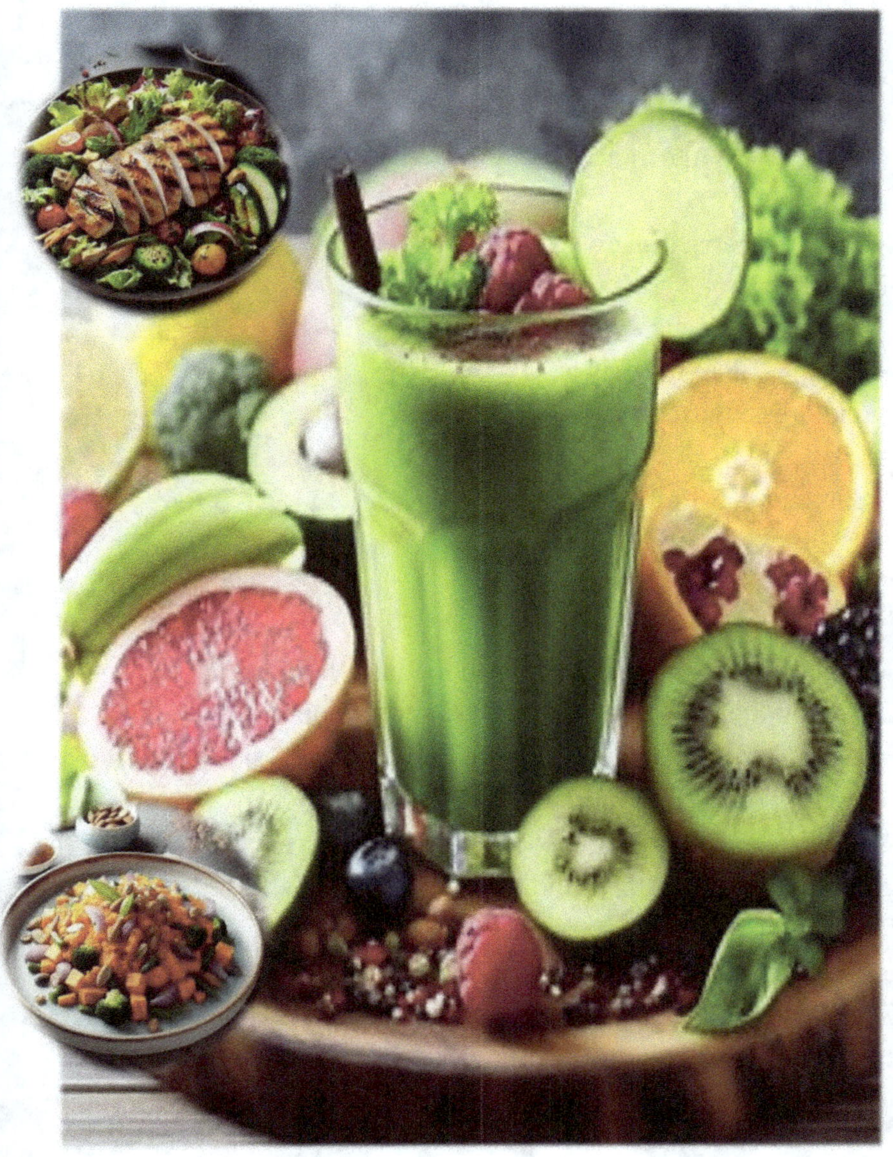

Grilled Chicken and Mixed Greens Salad

Prep Time:15 mins | **Cook Time: 15 mins** | **Servings: 1** | **Cal: 350**

Ingredients:

- 4 oz boneless, skinless chicken breast
- 2 cups mixed greens (spinach, arugula, and romaine)
- 1/4 cup cherry tomatoes, halved
- 1/4 cup cucumber, sliced
- 2 tbsp GERD-friendly salad dressing (recipe provided)
- Salt and pepper to taste

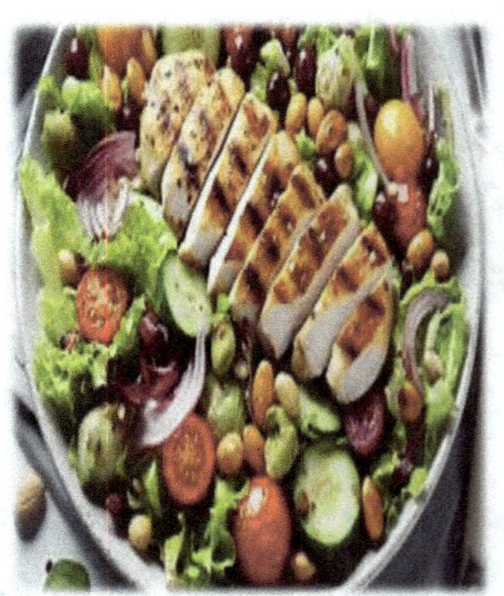

Instructions:

1. Preheat your grill or grill pan to medium-high heat.
2. Season the chicken breast with salt and pepper.
3. Grill the chicken for about 6-7 minutes per side until cooked through.
4. While the chicken is cooking, prepare your salad by mixing the greens, cherry tomatoes, and cucumber in a bowl.
5. Once the chicken is done, slice it into thin strips.
6. Arrange the sliced chicken on top of the salad.
7. Drizzle the GERD-friendly dressing over the salad and toss to coat evenly and enjoy your reflux-free grilled chicken salad!

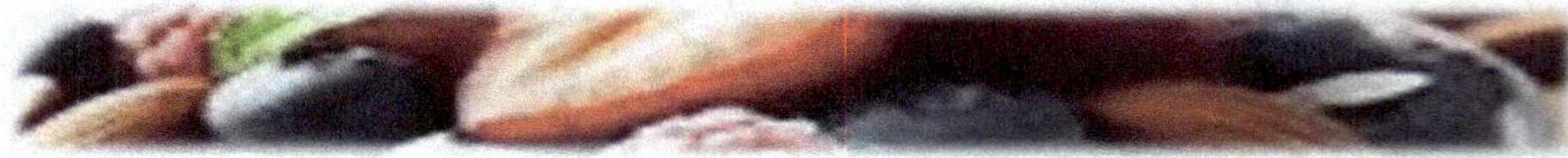

Quinoa and Black Bean Salad with Avocado Lime Dressing

Prep Time:20 mins | Cook Time: 15 mins | Servings: 1 | Cal: 450

Ingredients:

- 1/2 cup cooked quinoa

- 1/2 cup canned black beans, drained and rinsed

- 1/4 cup red bell pepper, diced

- 1/4 cup corn kernels (fresh or frozen)

- 1/4 cup fresh cilantro, chopped

- 1/2 ripe avocado, diced

- 1 tbsp olive oil

- Juice of 1 lime - Salt and pepper to taste

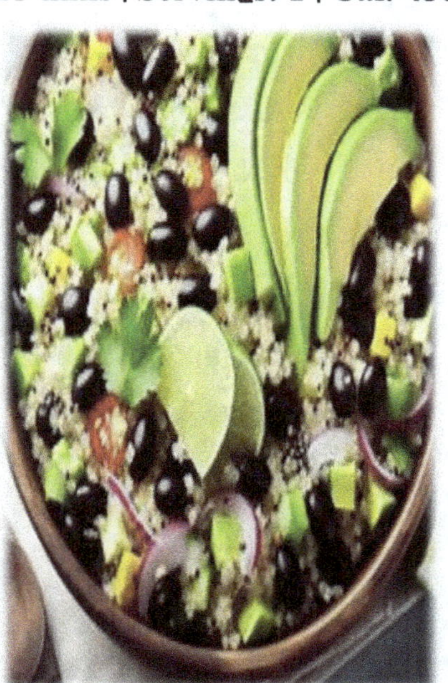

Instructions:

1. In a bowl, combine the cooked quinoa, black beans, red bell pepper, corn, and cilantro.

2. In a separate bowl, mash the diced avocado with lime juice, olive oil, salt, and pepper to create the dressing.

3. Add the avocado lime dressing to the salad and toss well.

4. Enjoy a delightful, nutrient-rich quinoa and black bean salad.

Spinach and Strawberry Salad with Balsamic Vinaigrette

Prep Time: 10 minutes │ Servings: 1 │ Calories: 280

Ingredients:

- 2 cups baby spinach

- 1 cup fresh strawberries, hulled and sliced

- 1/4 cup sliced almonds

- 2 tbsp balsamic vinaigrette dressing (GERD-friendly)

- Crumbled feta cheese (optional) and salt and pepper to taste

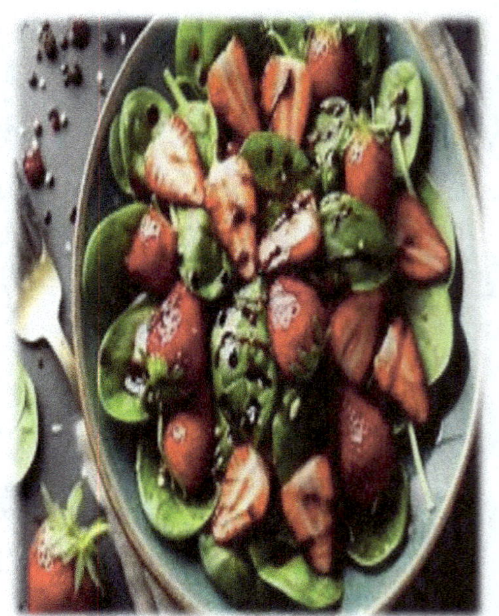

Instructions:

1. In a salad bowl, combine the baby spinach and sliced strawberries.

2. Sprinkle sliced almonds over the salad.

3. Drizzle the GERD-friendly balsamic vinaigrette dressing.

4. Optionally, add crumbled feta cheese for extra flavor.

5. Season with salt and pepper to taste and enjoy this delightful spinach and strawberry salad.

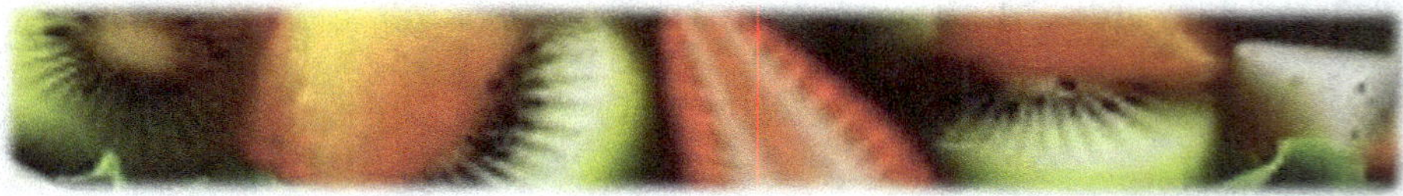

Tuna and White Bean Salad with Lemon Herb Dressing

Prep Time: 15 minutes | Servings: 1 | Calories: 430

Ingredients:

- 1 can (5 oz) tuna, drained

- 1 cup canned white beans, drained and rinsed

- 1/4 cup red onion, finely chopped

- 2 tbsp fresh parsley, chopped

- Juice of 1 lemon

- 2 tbsp olive oil

- Salt and pepper to taste

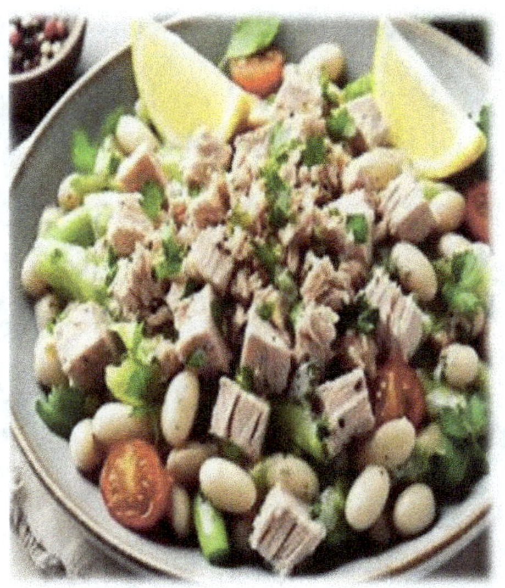

Instructions:

1. In a bowl, combine the tuna, white beans, chopped red onion, and fresh parsley.

2. In a separate bowl, whisk together lemon juice, olive oil, salt, and pepper to create the dressing.

3. Pour the lemon herb dressing over the salad and toss gently.

4. Savor this nutritious and satisfying tuna and white bean salad.

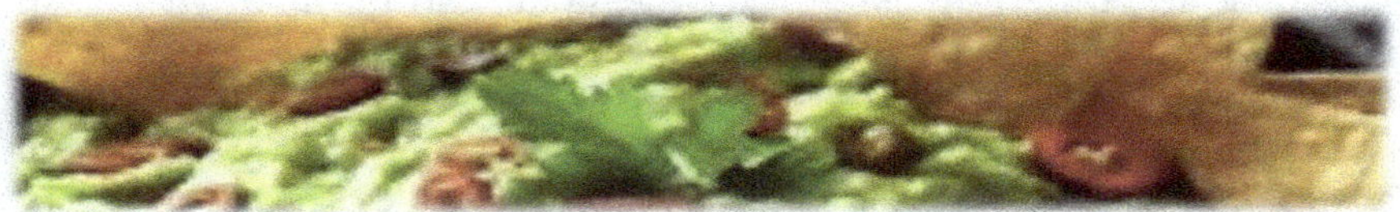

Roasted Veggie Quinoa Salad with Tahini Dressing

Prep Time: 20 mins | Cook Time:30 mins | Servings: 1 | Cal: 480

Ingredients:

- 1/2 cup cooked quinoa

- 1 cup mixed roasted vegetables (zucchini, bell peppers, carrots, etc.)

- 2 tbsp tahini

- 1 tbsp lemon juice

- 1 clove garlic, minced

- Salt and pepper to taste

- Fresh parsley for garnish

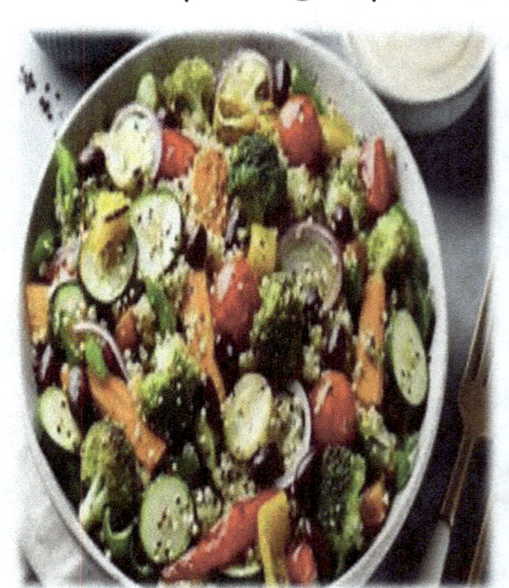

Instructions:

1. Preheat your oven to 400°F (200°C) and roast mixed vegetables with a drizzle of olive oil, salt, and pepper for about 30 minutes or until tender and slightly browned.

2. In a bowl, combine the cooked quinoa and roasted vegetables.

3. In a separate bowl, whisk together tahini, lemon juice, minced garlic, salt, and pepper to create the dressing.

4. Drizzle the tahini dressing over the salad and garnish with fresh parsley and enjoy a delectable roasted veggie quinoa salad.

Turkey and Avocado Wrap

Prep Time: 10 minutes | Servings: 1 | Calories: 400

Ingredients:

- 3 oz sliced turkey breast

- 1/2 avocado, sliced

- 1 whole-grain tortilla

- 1/4 cup baby spinach leaves

- 1 tbsp GERD-approved spread (recipe provided)

- Salt and pepper to taste

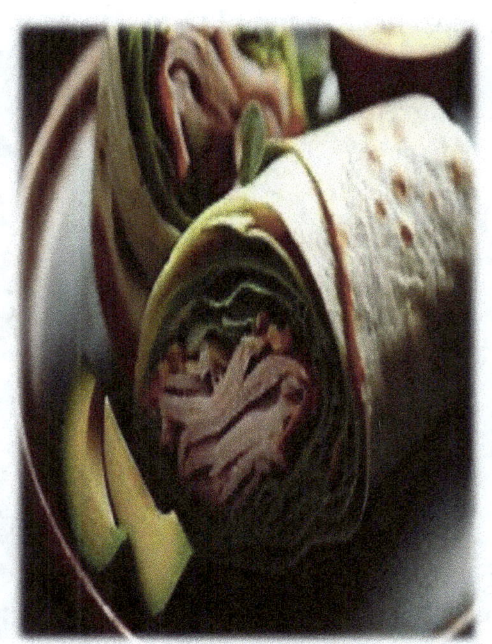

Instructions:

1. Lay the whole-grain tortilla flat and evenly spread the GERD-approved spread over it.

2. Layer the turkey slices, sliced avocado, and baby spinach leaves on top of the spread.

3. Season with salt and pepper to taste.

4. Roll up the tortilla, slice it in half, and enjoy your satisfying turkey and avocado wrap.

Hummus and Roasted Vegetable Sandwich

Prep Time: 20 mins | Cook Time: 30 mins | Servings:1 | Cal: 370

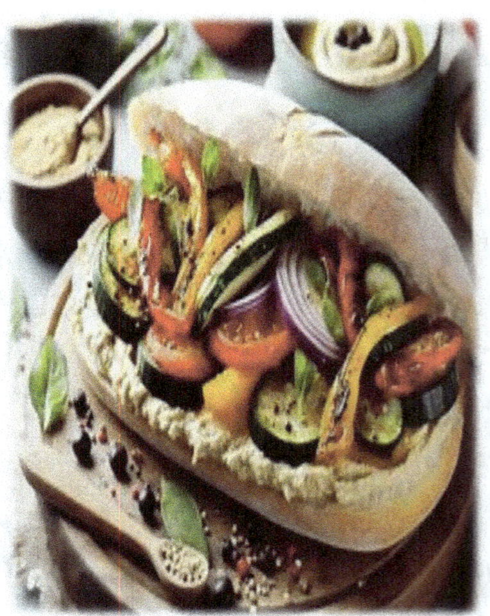

Ingredients:
- 2 slices whole-grain bread
- 2 tbsp hummus
- 1/2 cup mixed roasted vegetables (e.g., bell peppers, zucchini, and eggplant)
- 1/4 cup baby spinach leaves
- 1/4 cup red onion, thinly sliced
- Salt and pepper to taste

Instructions:

1. Roast the mixed vegetables in the oven at 400°F (200°C) for about 30 minutes or until tender.

2. Spread hummus on one slice of whole-grain bread.

3. Layer the roasted vegetables, baby spinach leaves, and red onion on the hummus-covered bread slice.

4. Season with salt and pepper to taste.

5. Top with the second slice of bread, slice the sandwich in half and enjoy your delightful hummus and roasted vegetable sandwich.

Smoked Salmon and Cucumber Wrap

Prep Time: 10 minutes | Servings: 1 | Calories: 300

Ingredients:

- 2 oz smoked salmon

- 1 whole-grain tortilla

- 1/4 cup cucumber, thinly sliced

- 2 tbsp GERD-approved spread (recipe provided)

- Fresh dill for garnish

- Salt and pepper to taste

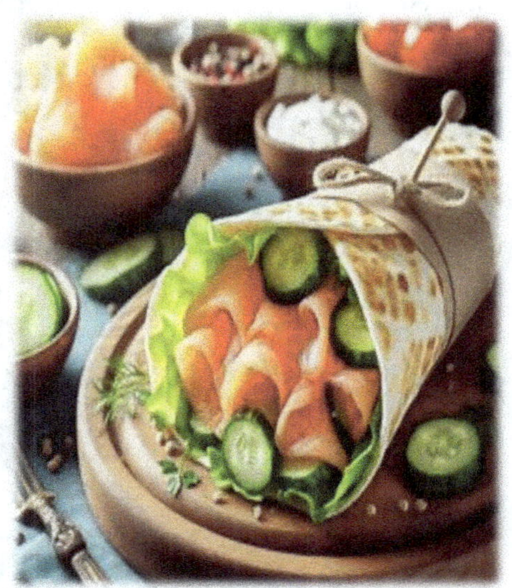

Instructions:

1. Lay the whole-grain tortilla flat and evenly spread the GERD-approved spread over it.

2. Layer the smoked salmon, thinly sliced cucumber, and fresh dill on top of the spread.

3. Season with salt and pepper to taste.

4. Roll up the tortilla, slice in half, and enjoy your refreshing smoked salmon and cucumber wrap.

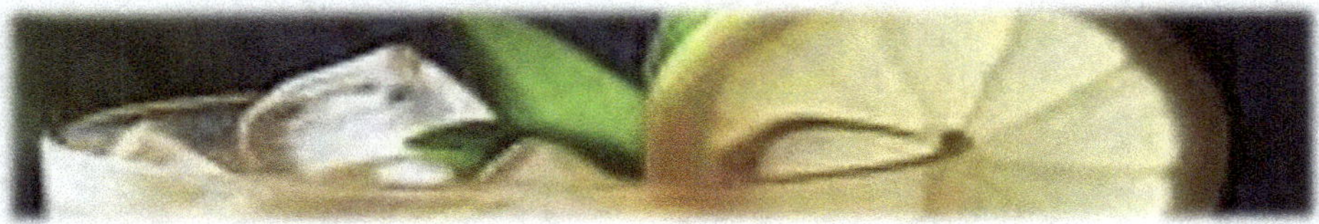

Caprese Panini with Pesto Spread

Prep Time:15 mins | Cook Time:10 mins | Servings:1 | Cal: 450

Ingredients:

- 2 slices whole-grain bread

- 2 oz fresh mozzarella cheese, sliced

- 1/2 ripe tomato, sliced

- Fresh basil leaves

- 1 tbsp pesto spread (GERD-friendly)

- Salt and pepper to taste

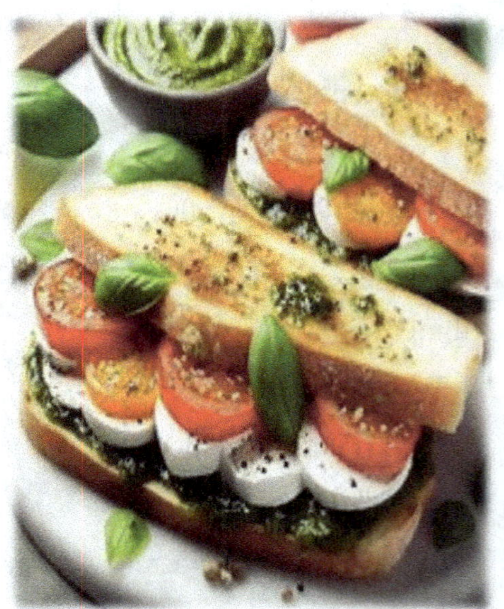

Instructions:

1. Spread the GERD-friendly pesto on one slice of whole-grain bread.

2. Layer the fresh mozzarella slices, tomato slices, and fresh basil leaves on top of the pesto.

3. Season with salt and pepper to taste.

4. Top with the second slice of bread and grill the sandwich in a Panini press or on the stovetop until it is golden brown and the cheese is melted.

5. Slice the Panini in half, and savor your gourmet Cap rese Panini with Pesto Spread.

Turkey and Cranberry Sandwich with Creamy Spread

Prep Time: 10 minutes | Servings: 1 | Calories: 400

Ingredients:

- 3 oz sliced turkey breast

- 2 slices whole-grain bread

- 2 tbsp cranberry sauce (GERD-friendly)

- 1 tbsp GERD-approved creamy spread (recipe provided)

- Fresh spinach leaves

- Salt and pepper to taste

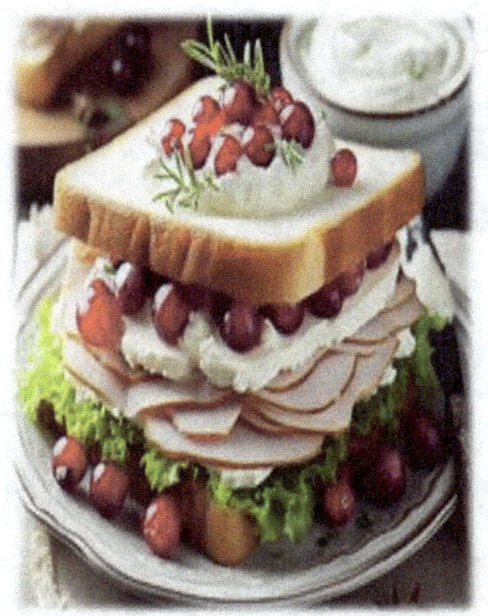

Instructions:

1. Spread the GERD-approved creamy spread on one slice of whole-grain bread.

2. Spread cranberry sauce on the second slice of bread.

3. Layer the turkey slices and fresh spinach leaves on top of the creamy spread-covered bread slice.

4. Season with salt and pepper to taste.

5. Top with the second slice of bread, slice the sandwich in half and enjoy your satisfying Turkey and Cranberry Sandwich.

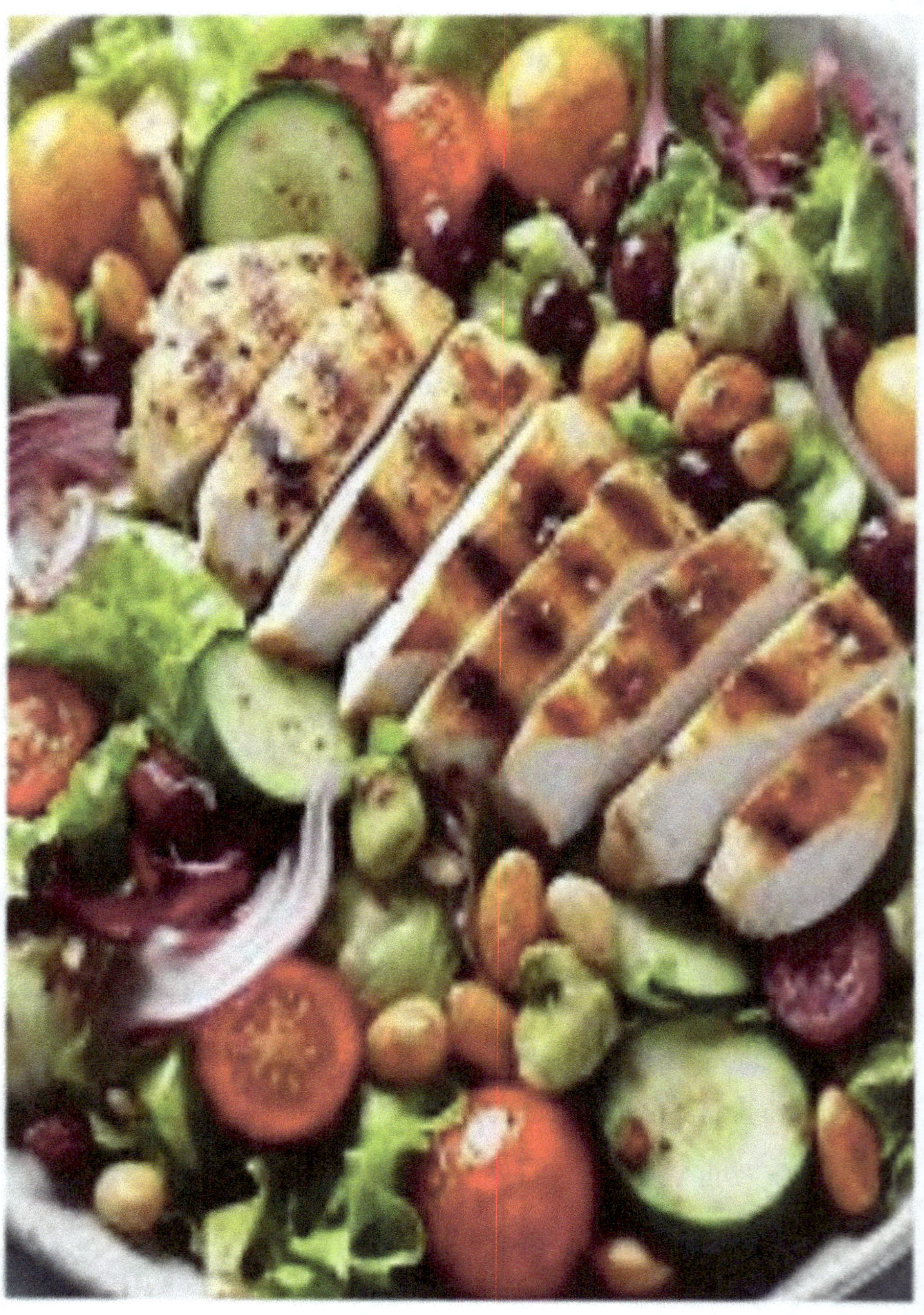

DELIGHTFUL DINNER RECIPES

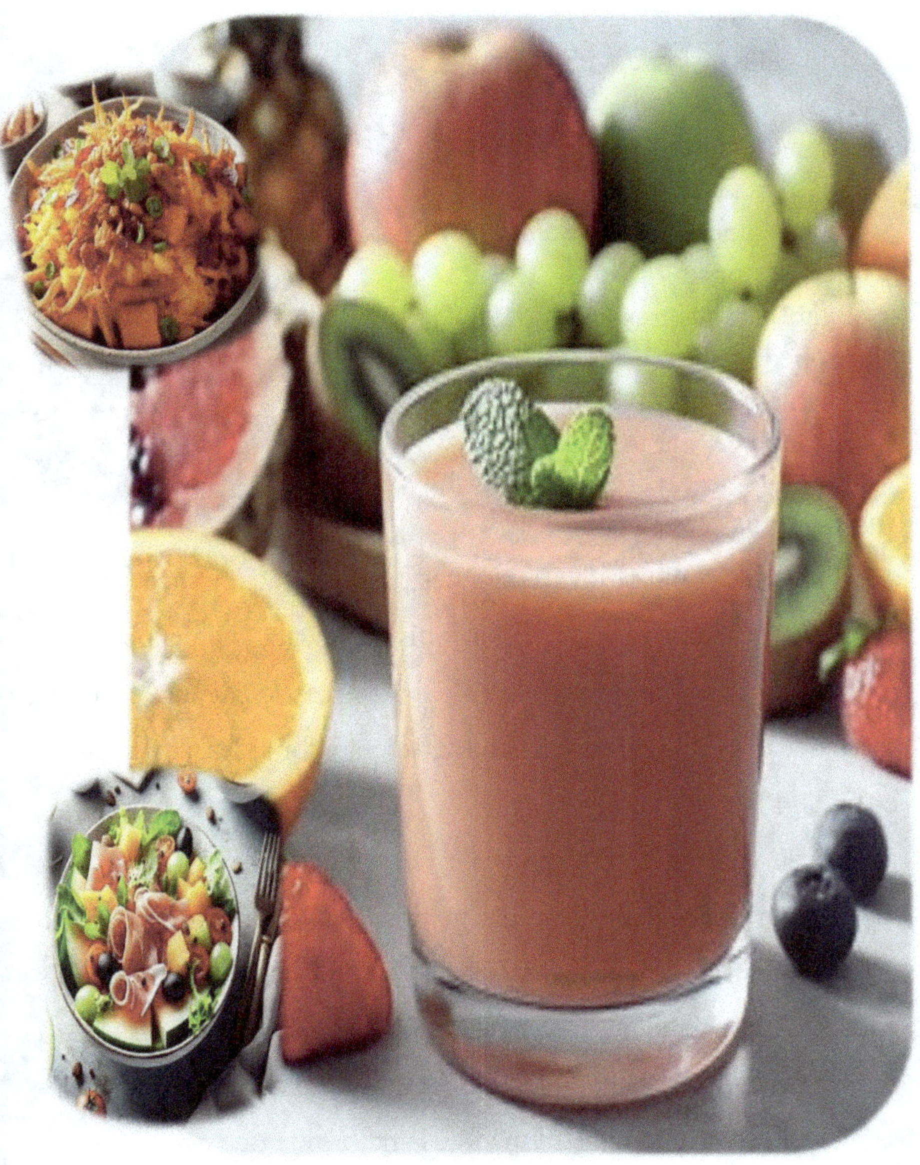

Grilled Lemon Herb Chicken

Prep Time: 15 mins │ Cook Time: 20 mins │ Servings: 1 │ Cal: 350

Ingredients:
- 1 boneless, skinless chicken breast
- 1 lemon, zested and juiced
- 2 cloves garlic, minced
- 2 tablespoons fresh rosemary, finely chopped
- 2 tablespoons fresh thyme, finely chopped
- 2 tablespoons olive oil
- Salt and pepper to taste

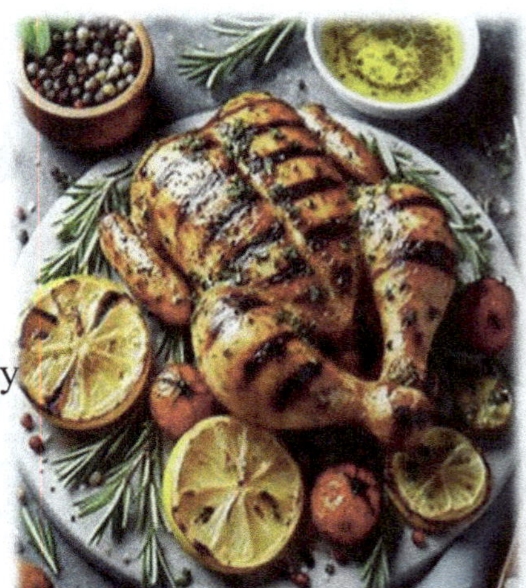

Instructions:

1. In a bowl, combine the lemon zest, lemon juice, minced garlic, chopped rosemary, chopped thyme, olive oil, salt, and pepper.

2. Place the chicken breast in a reseal able plastic bag and pour the marinade over it. Seal the bag and refrigerate for at least 30 minutes or up to 4 hours.

3. Preheat your grill to medium-high heat.

4. Remove the chicken from the marinade, allowing any excess to drip off. Grill the chicken for about 10 minutes per side or until it's cooked through and no longer pink in the center.

5. Serve the grilled lemon herb chicken with your choice of GERD-safe sides, such as steamed asparagus and brown rice.

Baked Salmon with Dill Sauce

Prep Time: 10 mins │ **Cook Time: 20 mins** │ **Servings: 1** │ **Cal: 300**

Ingredients:

- 1 salmon filet

- 1 tablespoon fresh dill, chopped

- 1 tablespoon Greek yogurt

- 1 clove garlic, minced

- 1 teaspoon lemon juice

- Salt and pepper to taste

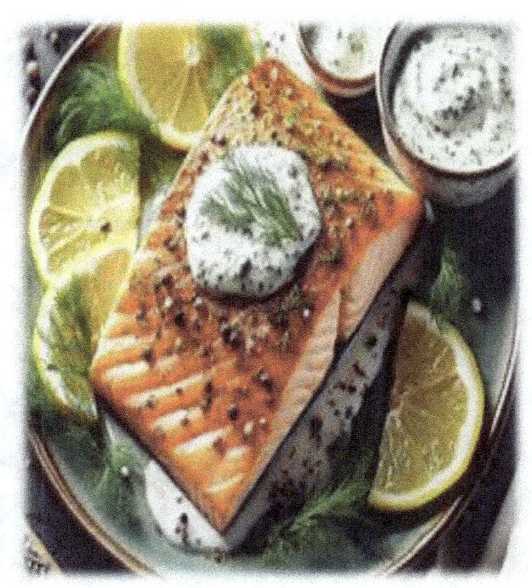

Instructions:

1. Preheat your oven to 350°F (175°C).

2. In a small bowl, mix the chopped dill, Greek yogurt, minced garlic, lemon juice, salt, and pepper.

3. Place the salmon filet on a baking sheet lined with parchment paper. Spread the dill sauce evenly on top of the salmon.

4. Bake in the preheated oven for 15-20 minutes or until the salmon flakes easily with a fork.

5. Serve the baked salmon with a side of steamed green beans and quinoa.

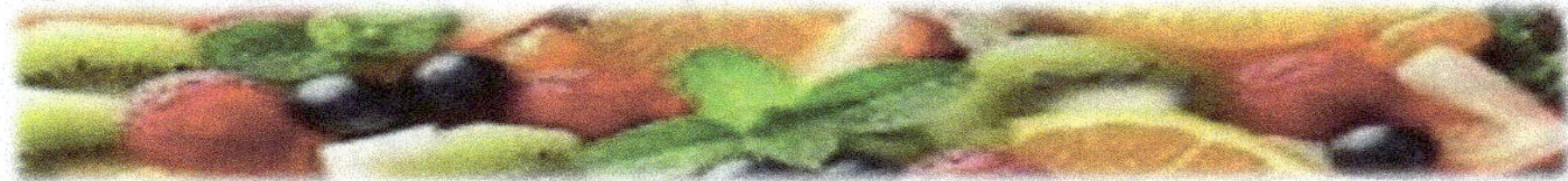

Turkey and Quinoa Stuffed Peppers

Prep Time: 20 mins │ Cook Time: 45 mins │ Servings: 1 │ Cal: 350

Ingredients:
- 2 bell peppers, any color
- 1/2 cup lean ground turkey
- 1/4 cup cooked quinoa
- 1/4 cup diced tomatoes
- 1/4 cup chopped spinach
- 1/4 cup low-sodium chicken broth
- 1/2 teaspoon Italian seasoning
- Salt and pepper to taste

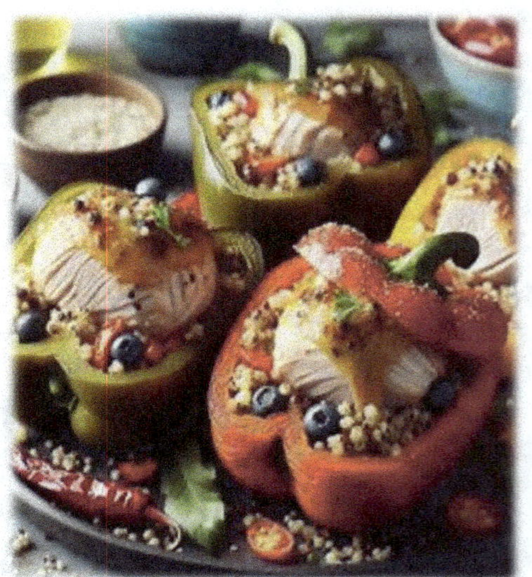

Instructions:
1. Preheat your oven to 375°F (190°C).
2. Cut the tops off the bell peppers and remove the seeds and membranes. Set aside.
3. In a skillet, cook the ground turkey until browned. Drain any excess fat.
4. In a bowl, combine the cooked turkey, quinoa, diced tomatoes, chopped spinach, Italian seasoning, salt, and pepper.
5. Stuff the bell peppers with the turkey and quinoa mixture.
6. Place the stuffed peppers in a baking dish and pour the chicken broth into the bottom of the dish.
7. Cover the dish with foil and bake for 35-40 minutes or until the peppers are tender. Serve the stuffed peppers with a side salad.

Quinoa and Vegetable Stir-Fry

Prep Time: 15 mins | Cook Time: 20 mins | Servings: 1 | Cal: 350

Ingredients:
- 1/2 cup cooked quinoa
- 1 cup mixed stir-fry vegetables (broccoli, bell peppers, snap peas, carrots)
- 2 tablespoons low-sodium soy sauce
- 1 tablespoon sesame oil
- 1 clove garlic, minced
- 1/2 teaspoon ginger, minced
- 1 tablespoon rice vinegar

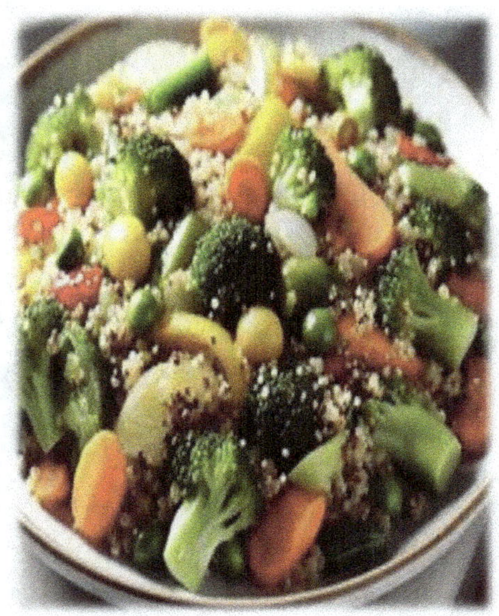

Instructions:

1. In a large skillet, heat the sesame oil over medium-high heat.

2. Add the minced garlic and ginger, and sauté for about 30 seconds, until fragrant.

3. Add the mixed stir-fry vegetables and stir-fry for 5-7 minutes, or until they are tender but still crisp.

4. In a small bowl, mix the low-sodium soy sauce and rice vinegar.

5. Add the cooked quinoa and the sauce to the skillet. Stir-fry for an additional 2-3 minutes.

6. Serve the Quinoa and Vegetable Stir-Fry immediately, garnished with sesame seeds if desired.

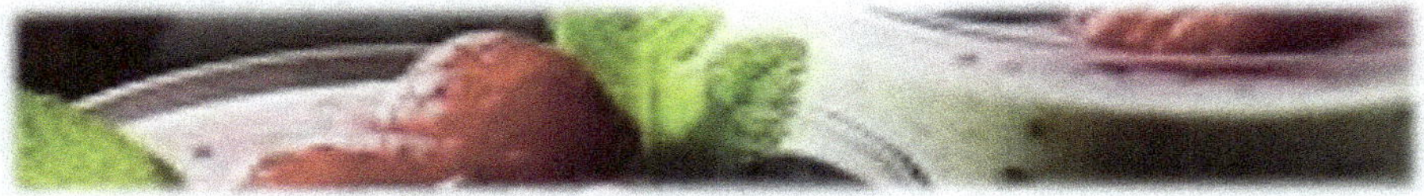

Zucchini Noodles with Pesto

Prep Time: 15 mins | Cook Time: 5 mins | Servings: 1 | Cal: 300

Ingredients:

- 2 medium zucchinis, spiralized into noodles
- 1/4 cup fresh basil leaves
- 2 tablespoons pine nuts
- 1/4 cup grated Parmesan cheese
- 1 clove garlic
- 3 tablespoons olive oil
- Salt and pepper to taste

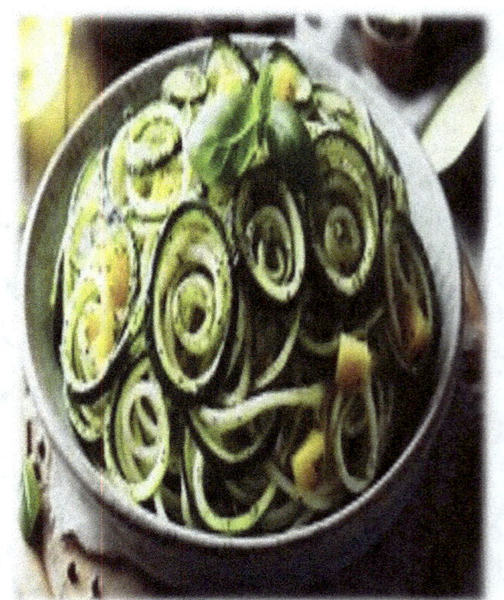

Instructions:

1. In a food processor, combine the basil leaves, pine nuts, Parmesan cheese, garlic, and olive oil. Blend until you have a smooth pesto sauce. Season with salt and pepper to taste.

2. Heat a large skillet over medium-high heat. Add the zucchini noodles and cook for about 3-5 minutes, tossing them occasionally until they are slightly tender.

3. Toss the zucchini noodles with the prepared pesto sauce.

4. Serve the Zucchini Noodles with Pesto as a light and flavorful dinner option.

Roasted Vegetable and Chickpea Salad

Prep Time: 15 mins | Cook Time: 25 mins | Servings: 1 | Cal: 400

Ingredients:
- 1 cup mixed roasted vegetables (zucchini, bell peppers, cherry tomatoes)
- 1/2 cup canned chickpeas, drained and rinsed
- 2 cups mixed greens
- 2 tablespoons balsamic vinaigrette
- 1/4 cup crumbled feta cheese
- Salt and pepper to taste

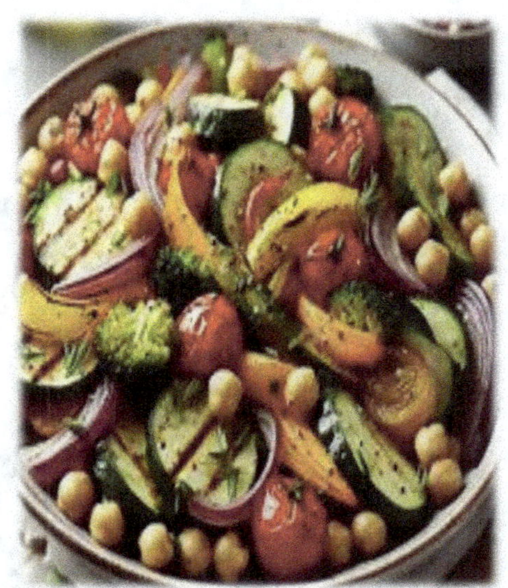

Instructions:

1. Preheat your oven to 400°F (200°C). Toss the mixed vegetables with olive oil, salt, and pepper, and roast for 20-25 minutes or until tender.

2. In a large bowl, combine the roasted vegetables, chickpeas, and mixed greens.

3. Drizzle the balsamic vinaigrette over the salad and toss to combine.

4. Top the salad with crumbled feta cheese and season with additional salt and pepper if desired.

5. Serve the Roasted Vegetable and Chickpea Salad as a hearty and GERD-friendly dinner.

Turkey and Spinach Stuffed Mushrooms

Prep Time: 20 mins | Cook Time: 25 mins | Servings:1 | Cal: 280

Ingredients:

- 4 large white mushrooms, stems removed
- 1/4 cup lean ground turkey
- 1/4 cup chopped fresh spinach
- 2 tablespoons low-fat cream cheese
- 1 clove garlic, minced
- 1/2 teaspoon Italian seasoning
- Salt and pepper to taste

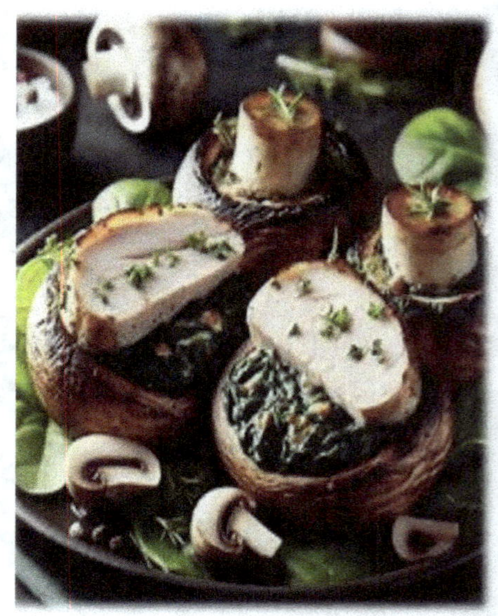

Instructions:

1. Preheat your oven to 375°F (190°C). Line a baking sheet with parchment paper.
2. In a skillet, cook the ground turkey until browned. Drain any excess fat.
3. In a bowl, combine the cooked turkey, chopped spinach, low-fat cream cheese, minced garlic, Italian seasoning, salt, and pepper.
4. Fill each mushroom cap with the turkey and spinach mixture.
5. Place the stuffed mushrooms on the prepared baking sheet and bake for 20-25 minutes or until the mushrooms are tender.
6. Serve the Turkey and Spinach Stuffed Mushrooms as a delightful dinner option.

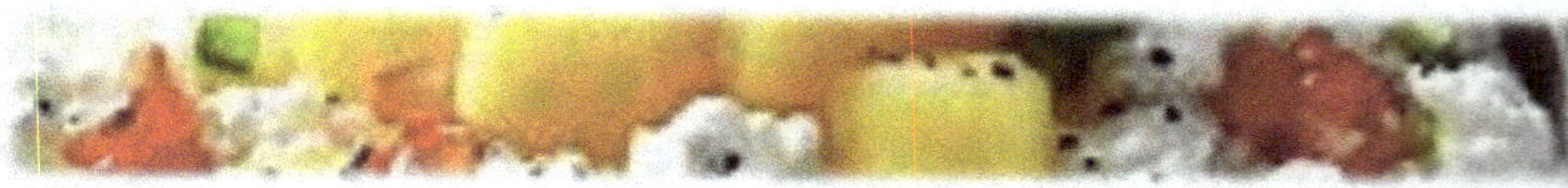

Brown Rice and Black Bean Bowl

Prep Time: 20 mins | Cook Time: 30 mins | Servings: 1 | Cal: 350

Ingredients:

- 1/2 cup cooked brown rice

- 1/2 cup canned black beans, drained and rinsed

- 1/2 cup diced red bell pepper

- 1/2 cup diced cucumber

- 1/4 cup fresh cilantro, chopped

- 2 tablespoons lime juice

- 1/2 teaspoon cumin

- Salt and pepper to taste

Instructions:

1. In a large bowl, combine the cooked brown rice, black beans, diced red bell pepper, diced cucumber, and chopped cilantro.

2. In a separate bowl, whisk together the lime juice, cumin, salt, and pepper.

3. Pour the dressing over the rice and bean mixture and toss to combine.

4. Serve the Brown Rice and Black Bean Bowl as a wholesome and satisfying dinner.

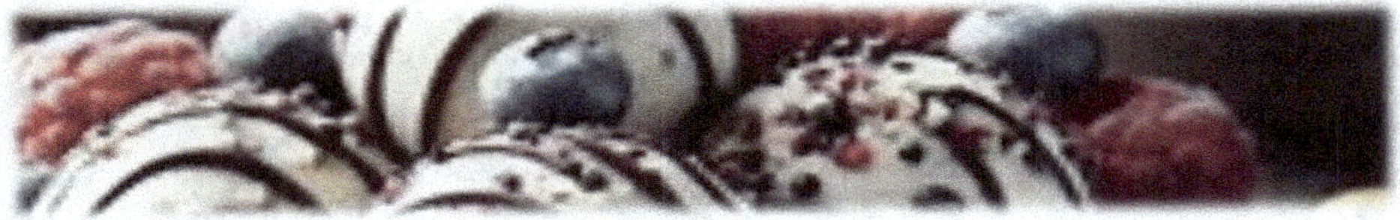

Baked Cod with Mediterranean Salsa

Prep Time: 15 mins | Cook Time: 20 mins | Servings: 1 | Cal: 320

Ingredients:

- 1 cod fillet

- 1/2 cup diced tomatoes

- 1/4 cup diced red onion

- 2 tablespoons fresh parsley, chopped

- 1 clove garlic, minced

- 1 tablespoon olive oil

- 1 tablespoon balsamic vinegar

- Salt and pepper to taste

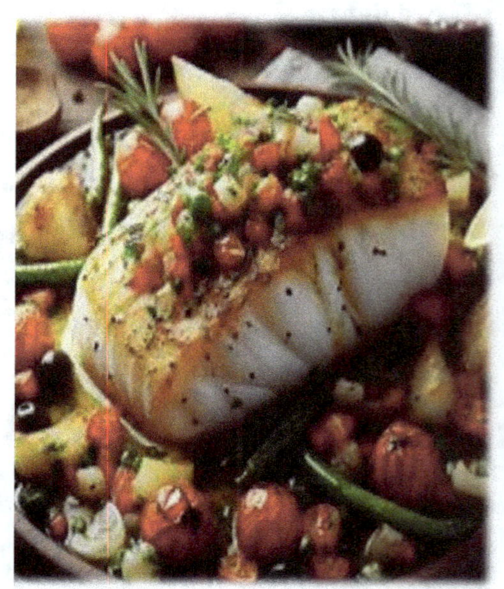

Instructions:

1. Preheat your oven to 375°F (190°C).

2. Place the cod filet on a baking sheet lined with parchment paper.

3. In a bowl, combine the diced tomatoes, diced red onion, chopped parsley, minced garlic, olive oil, balsamic vinegar, salt, and pepper.

4. Spoon the Mediterranean salsa over the cod fillet.

5. Bake in the preheated oven for 15-20 minutes or until the cod is opaque and flakes easily.

6. Serve the Baked Cod with Mediterranean Salsa as a refreshing and GERD-friendly dinner.

Eggplant Parmesan

Prep Time: 25 mins | Cook Time: 40 mins | Servings: 1 | Cal: 380

Ingredients:
- 1 small eggplant, sliced into rounds
- 1/2 cup marinara sauce (low-acid variety)
- 1/2 cup shredded mozzarella cheese
- 2 tablespoons grated Parmesan cheese
- 1/2 cup breadcrumbs (use gluten-free for GERD)
- 1/4 cup fresh basil leaves
- 2 tablespoons olive oil
- Salt and pepper to taste

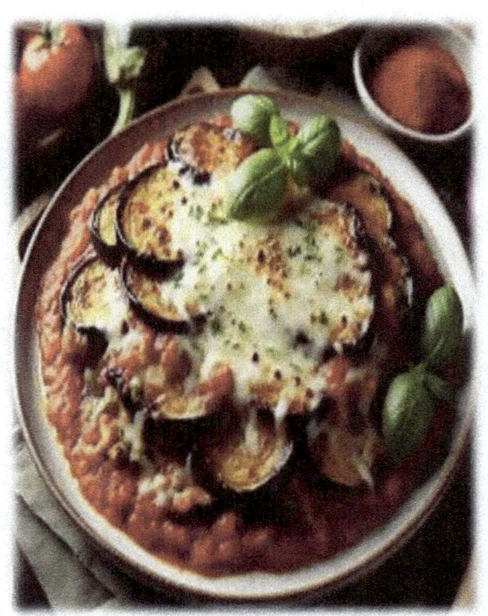

Instructions:
1. Preheat your oven to 375°F (190°C).
2. In a bowl, combine the breadcrumbs, grated Parmesan cheese, fresh basil leaves, olive oil, salt, and pepper.
3. Dip each eggplant slice into the breadcrumb mixture, coating both sides.
4. In a baking dish, layer the coated eggplant slices with marinara sauce and shredded mozzarella cheese.
5. Repeat the layers until all the eggplant slices are used.
6. Bake in the preheated oven for 30-40 minutes or until the cheese is bubbly and golden.
7. Serve the Eggplant Parmesan as a comforting and GERD-friendly dinner.

Lemon Garlic Shrimp and Asparagus

Prep Time: 15 mins │ Cook Time: 10 mins │ Servings: 1 │ Cal: 300

Ingredients:

- 6 large shrimp, peeled and deveined

- 1/2 bunch asparagus, trimmed

- 1 clove garlic, minced

- 1 lemon, zested and juiced

- 2 tablespoons olive oil

- 1/2 teaspoon red pepper flakes (optional)

- Salt and pepper to taste

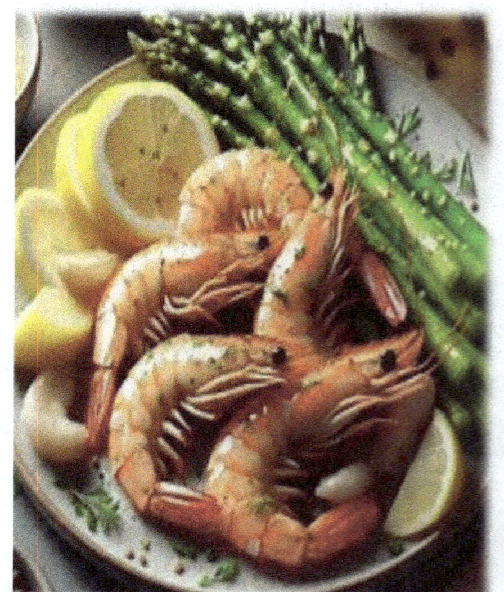

Instructions:

1. In a bowl, combine the minced garlic, lemon zest, lemon juice, olive oil, red pepper flakes (if using), salt, and pepper.

2. Toss the shrimp and asparagus in the prepared lemon garlic marinade.

3. Heat a skillet over medium-high heat. Add the shrimp and asparagus and cook for 2-3 minutes per side until the shrimp are pink and opaque.

4. Serve the Lemon Garlic Shrimp and Asparagus as a refreshing and GERD-friendly dinner.

REFRESHING SNACKS AND APPETIZERS RECIPES

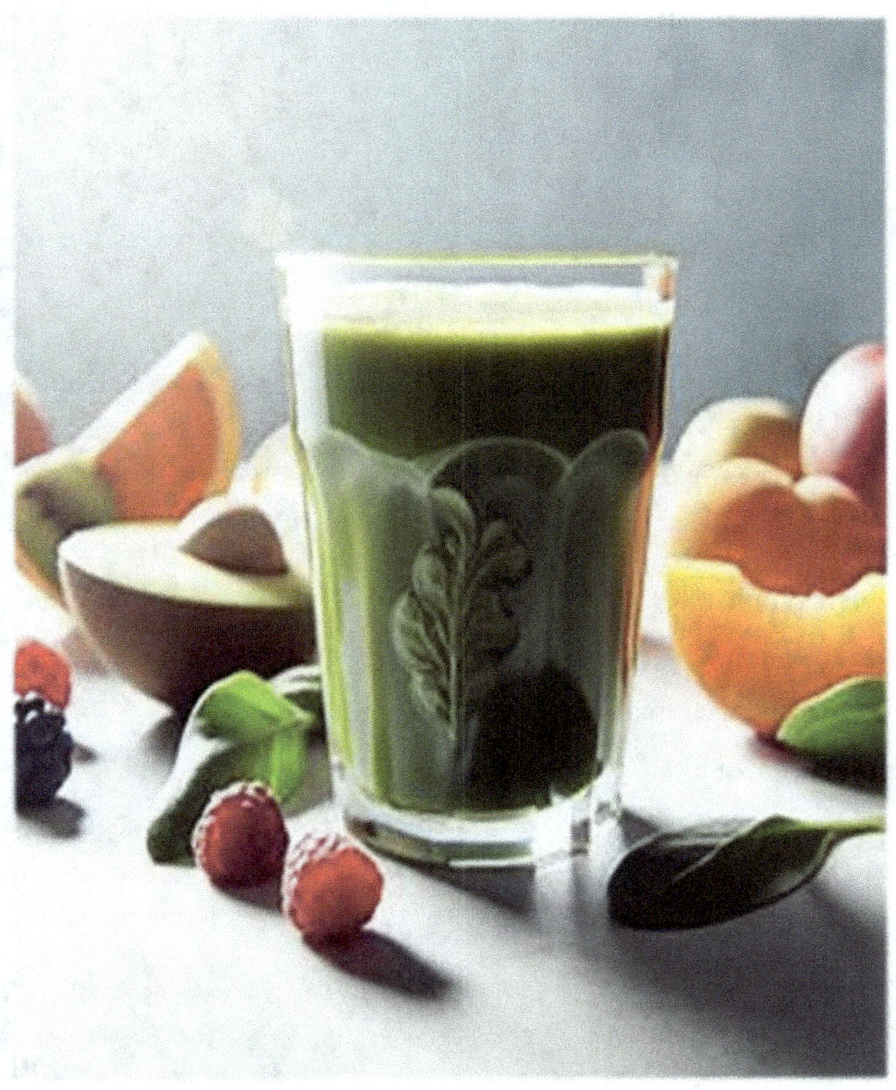

Greek Yogurt Tzatziki with Fresh Veggie Dippers

Prep Time: 10 mins | Servings: 1 | Calories: 100

Ingredients:

- 1/2 cup Greek yogurt

- 1/4 cucumber, grated and squeezed of excess moisture

- 1 clove garlic, minced

- 1 tbsp fresh dill, chopped

- Juice of 1/2 lemon

- Salt and pepper to taste

- Fresh vegetable dippers (carrots, cucumbers, bell peppers, etc.)

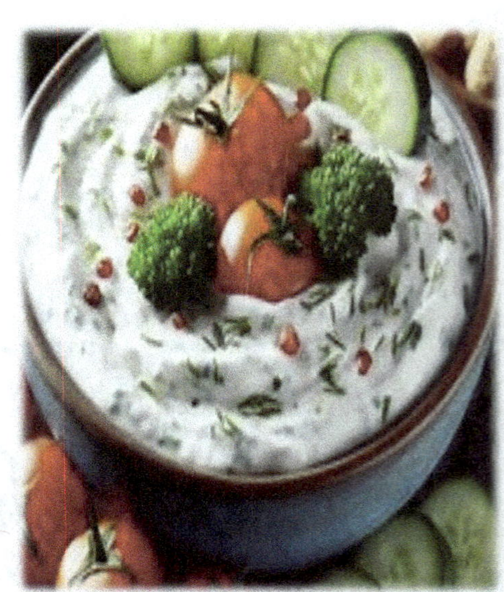

Instructions:

1. In a bowl, combine Greek yogurt, grated cucumber, minced garlic, chopped fresh dill, and lemon juice.

2. Season with salt and pepper to taste.

3. Serve the Tzatziki dip with a colorful array of fresh vegetable dippers.

4. Enjoy a refreshing and guilt-free snack.

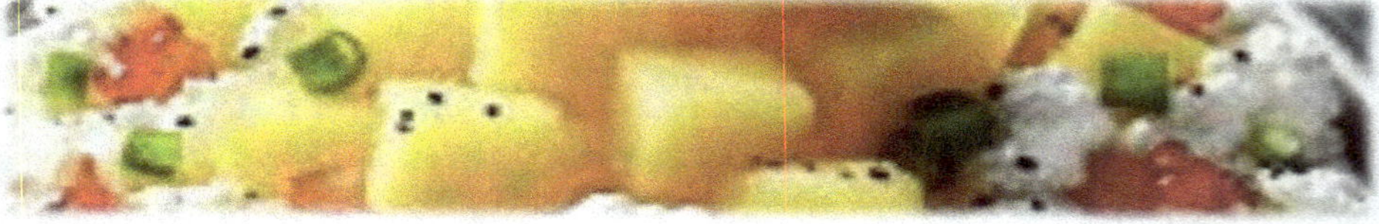

Baked Sweet Potato Chips

Prep Time: 15 mins | Cook Time: 20 mins | Servings:1 | Cal: 100

Ingredients:

- 2 sweet potatoes, thinly sliced
- 1 tbsp olive oil
- 1/2 tsp paprika
- 1/2 tsp garlic powder
- Salt and pepper to taste

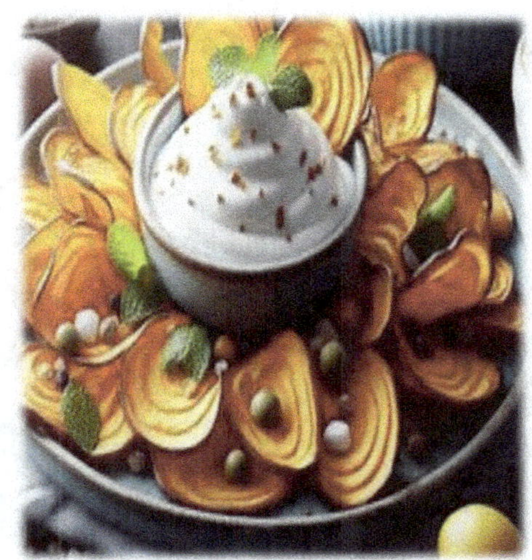

Instructions:

1. Preheat your oven to 375°F (190°C) and line a baking sheet with parchment paper.

2. In a bowl, toss the thinly sliced sweet potatoes with olive oil, paprika, garlic powder, salt, and pepper.

3. Arrange the seasoned sweet potato slices on the baking sheet in a single layer.

4. Bake for about 20 minutes, flipping the slices halfway through until they are golden and crispy.

5. Allow them to cool, and then enjoy your guilt-free Baked Sweet Potato Chips.

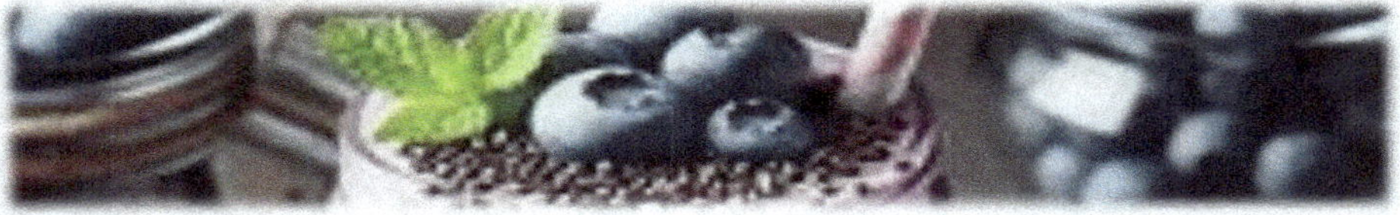

Avocado Hummus with Whole Wheat Pita Chips

Prep Time: 10 mins | Cook Time: 10 mins | Servings: 1 | Cal: 250

Ingredients:

- 1/2 avocado

- 1/2 cup canned chickpeas, drained and rinsed

- 1 clove garlic

- Juice of 1 lime

- 2 tbsp tahini

- 2 tbsp water

- Salt and pepper to taste

- Whole wheat pita chips

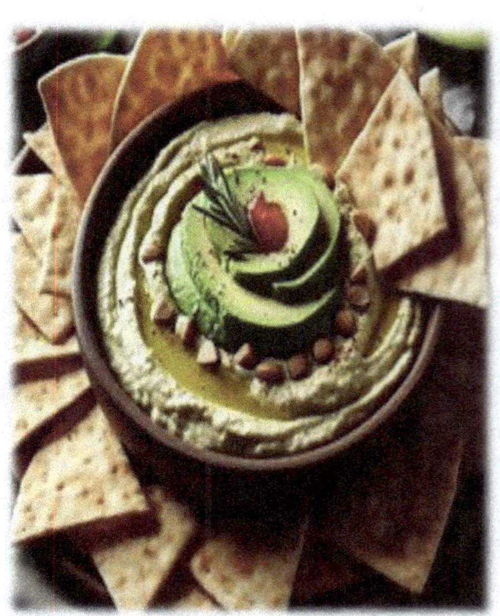

Instructions:

1. In a food processor, blend the avocado, chickpeas, garlic, lime juice, tahini, water, salt, and pepper until smooth.

2. Serve the Avocado Hummus with whole wheat pita chips.

3. Enjoy this creamy and nutritious snack.

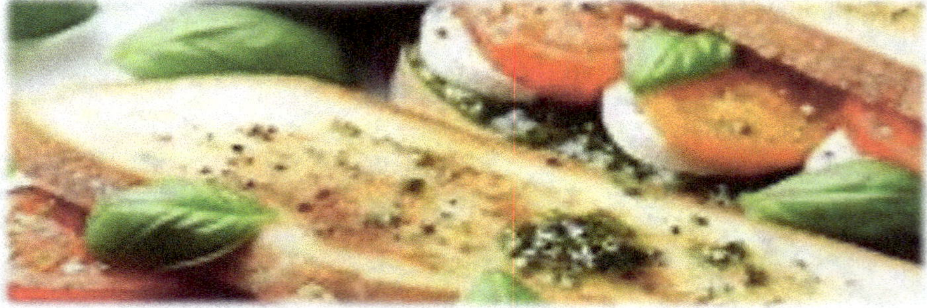

Guacamole with Baked Tortilla Chips

Prep Time: 15 mins | Cook Time: 10 mins | Servings: 1 | Cal: 250

Ingredients:

- 2 ripe avocados

- 1/4 cup red onion, finely chopped

- 1/4 cup tomato, diced

- 2 tbsp fresh cilantro, chopped

- Juice of 1 lime

- Salt and pepper to taste

- Whole wheat tortilla chips (recipe provided)

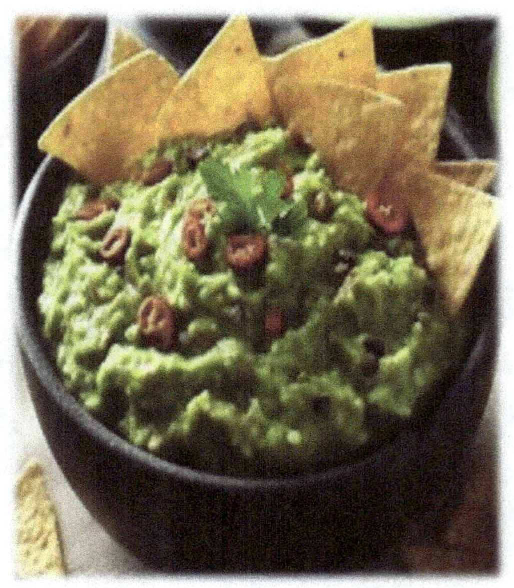

Instructions:

1. In a bowl, mash the ripe avocados with a fork.

2. Add finely chopped red onion, diced tomato, chopped fresh cilantro, lime juice, salt, and pepper. Mix until well combined.

3. Serve the Guacamole with baked whole wheat tortilla chips.

4. Enjoy this classic and healthy snack.

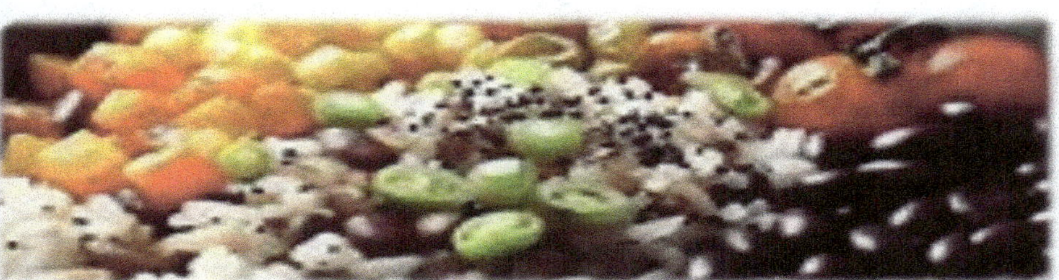

Whole Wheat Tortilla Chips

Prep Time: 10 mins | Cook Time: 10 mins | Servings: 1 | Cal: 100

Ingredients:

- 2 whole wheat tortillas

- 1 tsp olive oil

- 1/2 tsp paprika

- Salt to taste

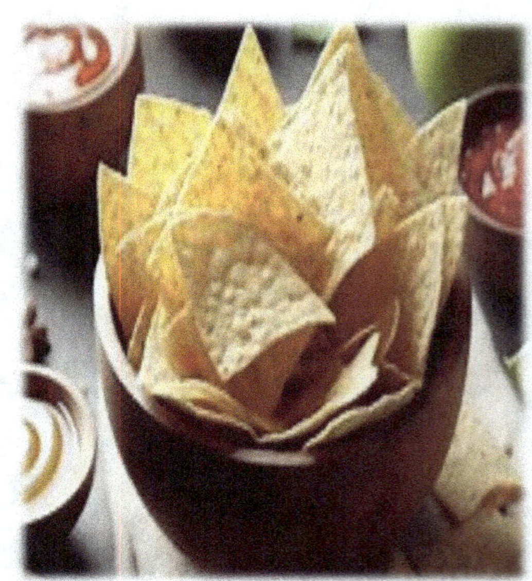

Instructions:

1. Preheat your oven to 350°F (175°C) and line a baking sheet with parchment paper.

2. Brush the whole wheat tortillas with olive oil and sprinkle with paprika and salt.

3. Slice the tortillas into wedges or strips.

4. Arrange the seasoned tortilla slices on the baking sheet in a single layer.

5. Bake for about 10 minutes until they're golden and crispy.

6. Allow them to cool, and then serve with your favorite dips.

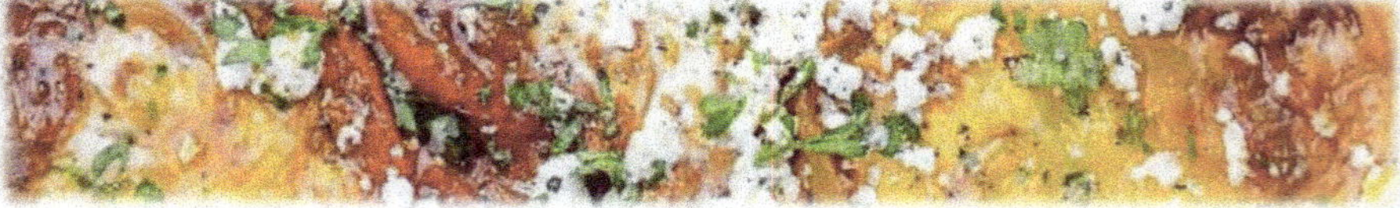

Almond and Berry Protein Balls

Prep Time: 10 mins | Servings: 1 | Cal: 90

Ingredients:

- 1/4 cup almonds

- 1/4 cup dried mixed berries (e.g., cranberries, blueberries)

- 1/2 tbsp of vanilla protein powder

- 1/4 tbsp honey

- 1/4 tsp vanilla extract

- Pinch of salt

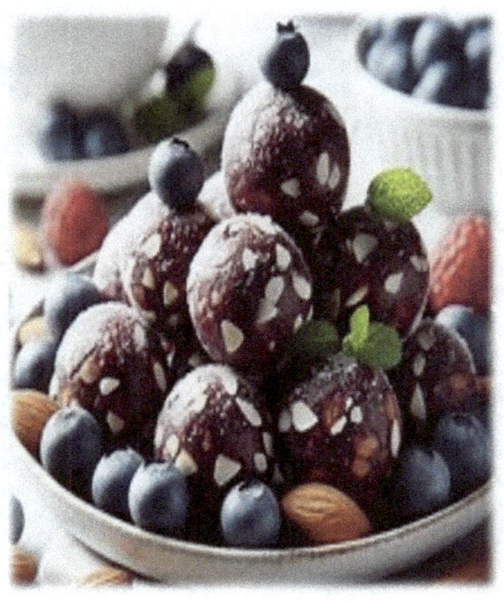

Instructions:

1. In a food processor, blend almonds until finely chopped.

2. Add dried mixed berries, protein powder, honey, vanilla extract, and a pinch of salt. Continue blending until the mixture comes together.

3. Roll the mixture into small balls and place them on a tray.

4. Chill in the refrigerator for about 30 minutes before enjoying these Almond and Berry Protein Balls.

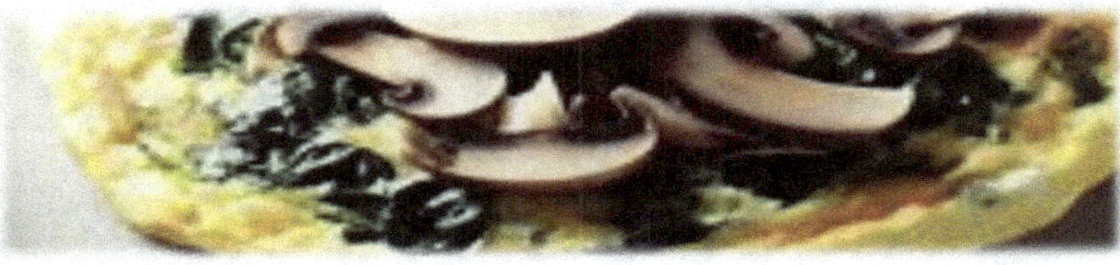

Edamame with Chili-Lime Seasoning

Prep Time: 5 mins | Cook Time: 5 mins | Servings: 1 | Cal: 90

Ingredients:

- 2 cups frozen edamame, thawed

- 1 tbsp olive oil

- 1/2 tsp chili powder

- Zest and juice of 1 lime

- Salt to taste

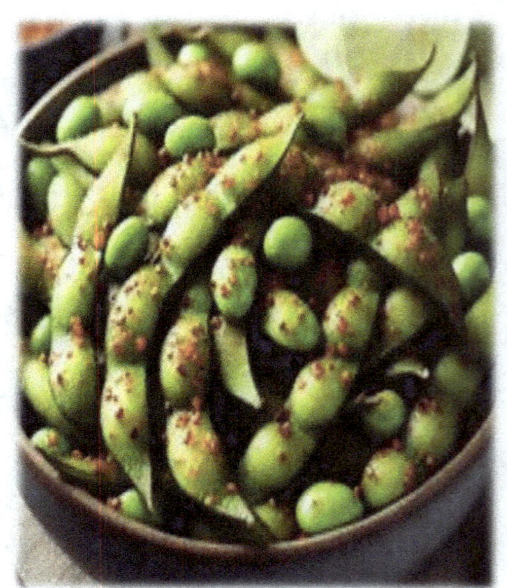

Instructions:

1. Heat olive oil in a pan and add the thawed edamame.

2. Sauté for about 5 minutes until they're heated through.

3. Remove from heat and sprinkle with chili powder, lime zest, lime juice, and salt.

4. Toss well and enjoy this zesty Edamame with Chili-Lime Seasoning.

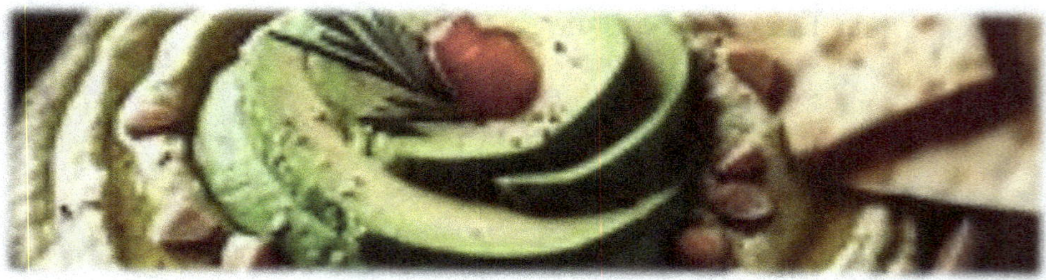

Cottage Cheese and Pineapple Salsa

Prep Time: 5 mins | Servings: 1 | Cal: 200

Ingredients:

- 1/2 cup low-fat cottage cheese

- 1/2 cup fresh pineapple, diced

- 1/4 cup red bell pepper, diced

- 1/4 cup red onion, finely chopped

- 1/2 jalapeño pepper, finely chopped (optional for spice)

- Fresh cilantro for garnish

- Salt and pepper to taste

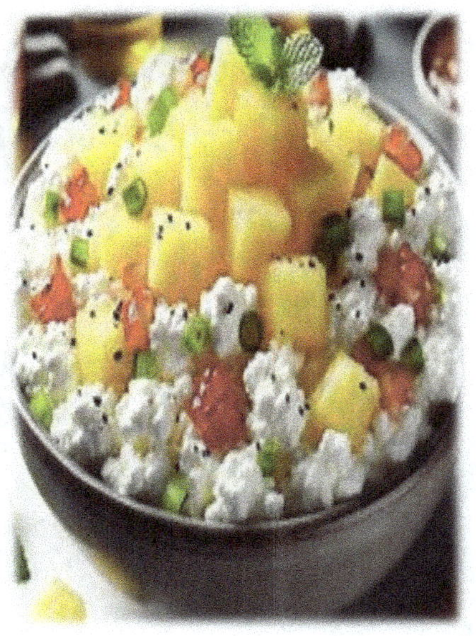

Instructions:

1. In a bowl, combine low-fat cottage cheese, fresh pineapple, diced red bell pepper, finely chopped red onion, and optional jalapeño pepper.

2. Season with salt and pepper to taste.

3. Garnish with fresh cilantro.

4. Enjoy this quick and satisfying Cottage Cheese and Pineapple Salsa.

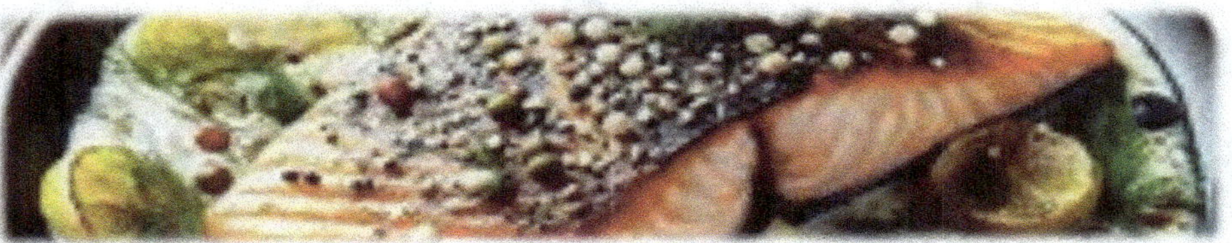

Cucumber and Hummus Bites

Prep Time: 10 mins | Servings: 1 | Calories: 50

Ingredients:

- 1 cucumber

- 1/2 cup hummus

(GERD-friendly)

- Fresh dill for garnish

- Paprika for garnish

- Salt and pepper to taste

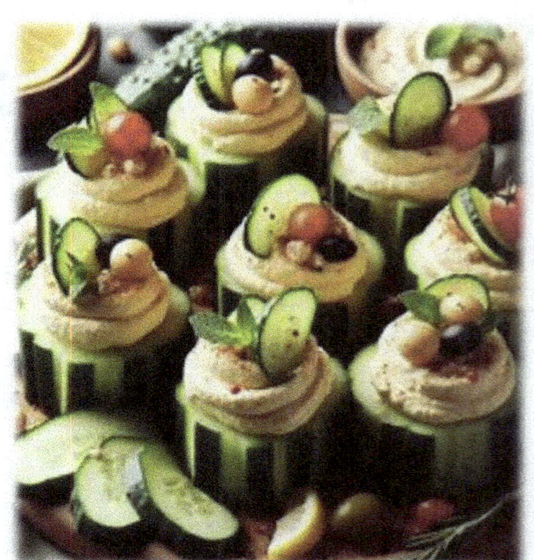

Instructions:

1. Slice the cucumber into rounds.

2. Spread a dollop of GERD-friendly hummus on each cucumber slice.

3. Garnish with fresh dill and a sprinkle of paprika.

4. Season with salt and pepper to taste.

5. Enjoy these refreshing Cucumber and Hummus Bites.

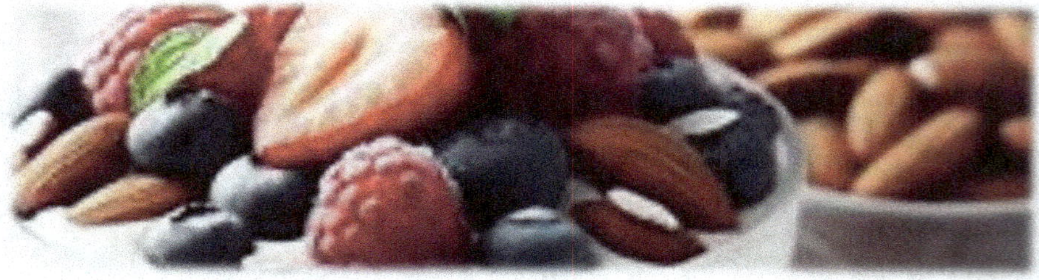

Baked Zucchini Fries with Garlic Aioli

Prep Time: 15 mins | Cook Time: 20 mins | Servings: 1 | Cal: 60

Ingredients:

- 2 zucchinis, cut into fries

- 1/2 cup whole wheat breadcrumbs

- 1/4 cup grated Parmesan cheese

- 1/2 tsp garlic powder
- 1/2 tsp dried oregano
- Salt and pepper to taste
- Cooking spray
- Garlic aioli (recipe provided)

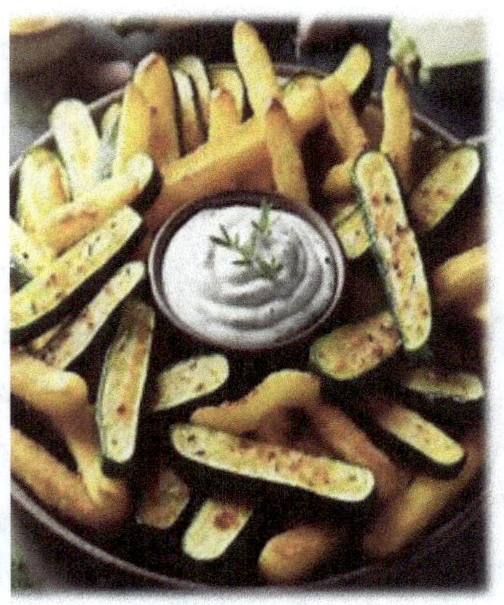

Instructions:

1. Preheat your oven to 425°F (220°C) and line a baking sheet with parchment paper.

2. In a bowl, combine whole wheat breadcrumbs, grated Parmesan cheese, garlic powder, dried oregano, salt, and pepper.

3. Dip the zucchini fries in the breadcrumb mixture, ensuring they're coated evenly.

4. Place the coated zucchini fries on the baking sheet and lightly spray with cooking spray.

5. Bake for about 20 minutes until they're golden and crispy.

6. Serve with the Garlic Aioli for dipping.

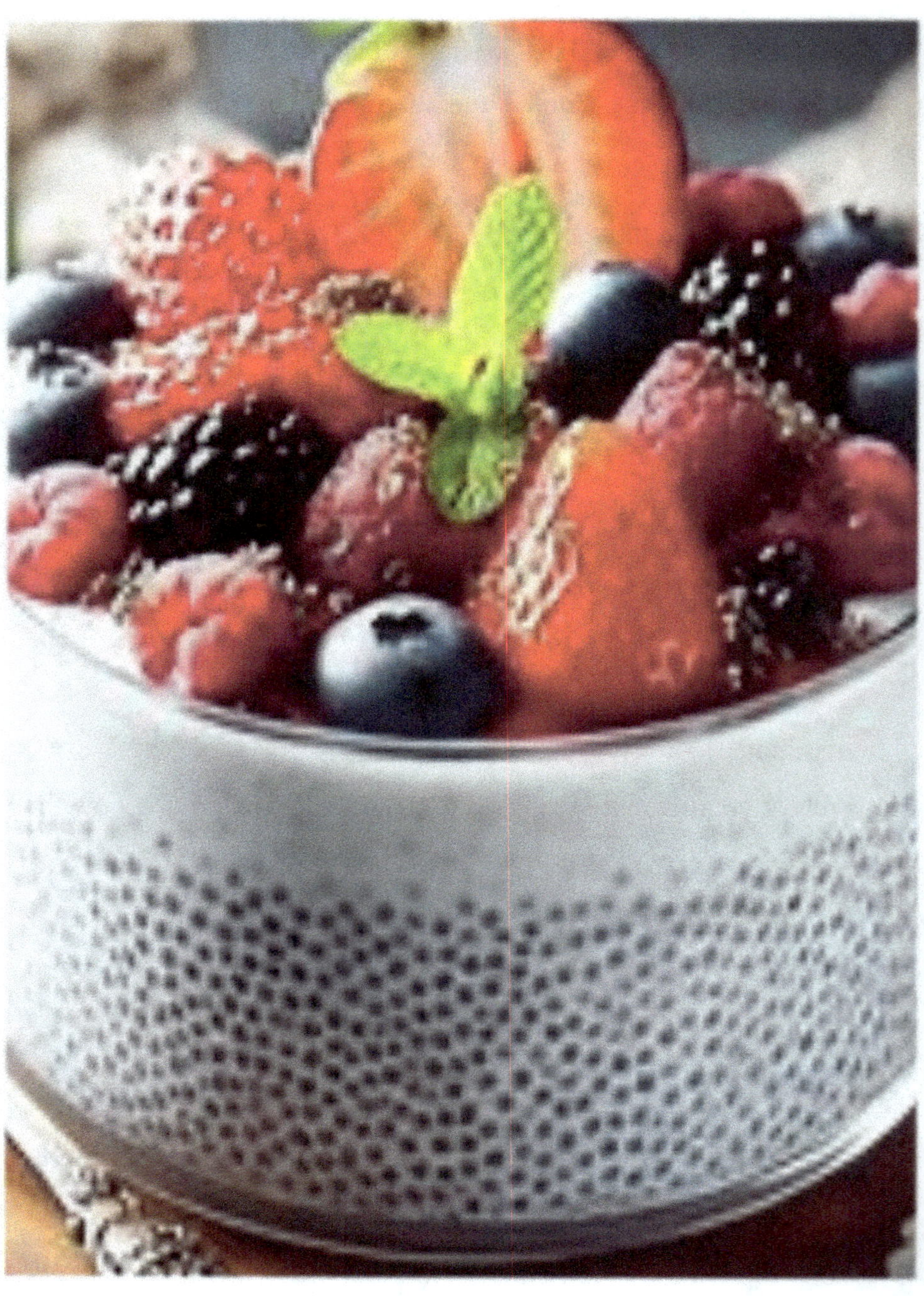

LUSCIOUS DESSERT RECIPES

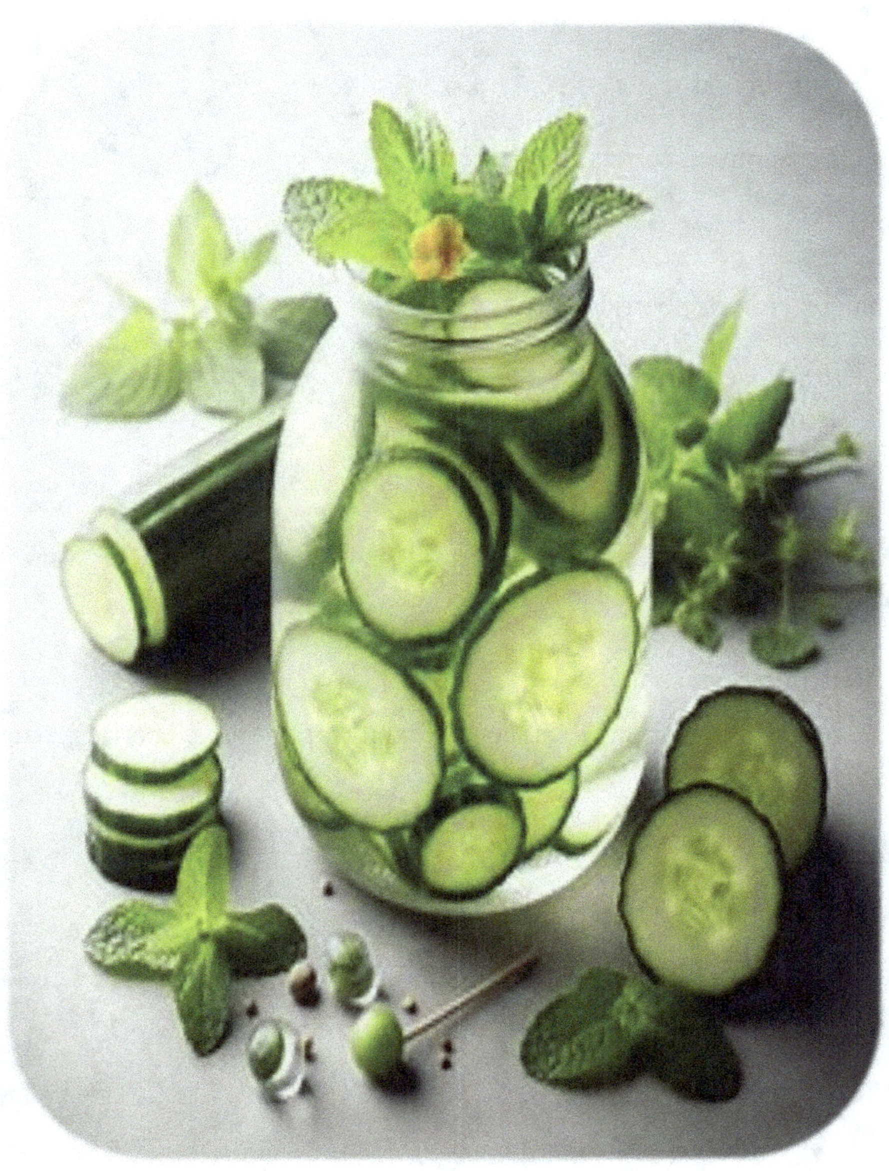

Almond and Berry Parfait

Prep Time: 10 mins │ Servings: 1 │ Cal: 250

Ingredients:

- 1 cup almond yogurt

- 1/2 cup mixed berries

(e.g., strawberries,

blueberries, raspberries)

- 1 tbsp sliced almonds

- 1 tsp honey (optional)

- Fresh mint leaves for

garnish

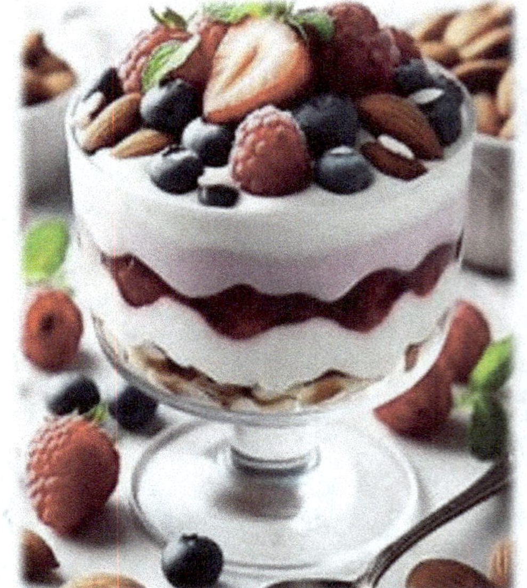

Instructions:

1. In a glass or serving dish, layer almond yogurt, mixed berries, and sliced almonds.

2. Drizzle with honey if desired.

3. Garnish with fresh mint leaves.

4. Enjoy this luscious Almond and Berry Parfait.

Chia Seed Pudding with Mango

Prep Time: 10 mins (plus chilling time) | Servings: 1 | Cal: 200

Ingredients:

- 3 tbsp chia seeds
- 1 cup unsweetened almond milk
- 1/2 cup fresh mango, diced
- 1/2 tsp vanilla extract
- 1 tsp honey (optional)

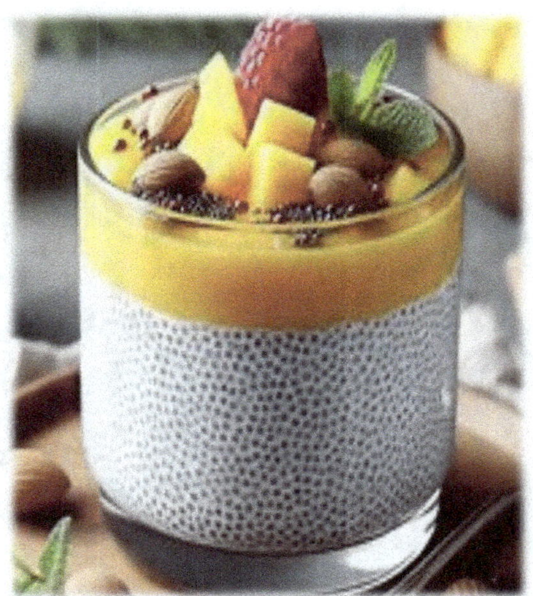

Instructions:

1. In a bowl, combine chia seeds, unsweetened almond milk, and vanilla extract.

2. Stir well and let it sit in the refrigerator for at least 2 hours or overnight until it thickens.

3. Layer chia seed pudding with diced mango.

4. Drizzle with honey if desired.

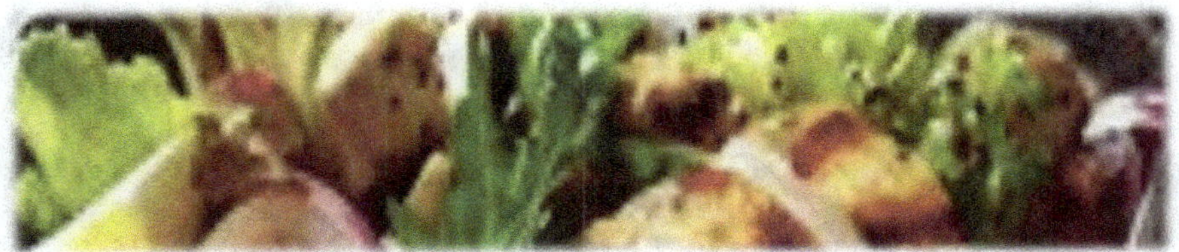

Cinnamon and Banana Oatmeal

Prep Time: 5 mins | Cook Time: 10 mins | Servings: 1 | Cal: 250

Ingredients:

- 1/2 cup old-fashioned oats

- 1 cup unsweetened almond milk

- 1 ripe banana, sliced

- 1/2 tsp ground cinnamon

- 1 tsp honey (optional)

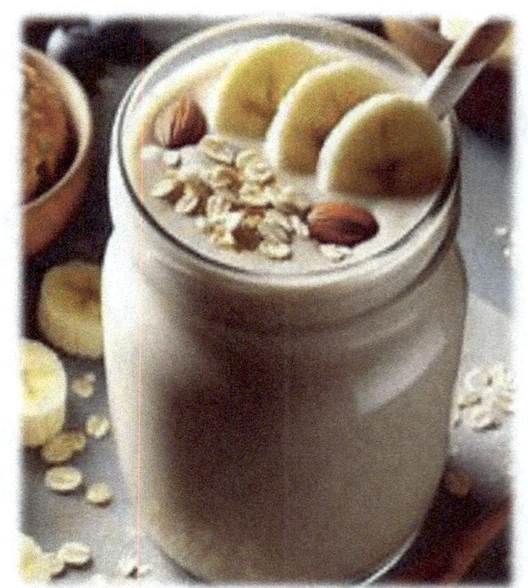

Instructions:

1. In a saucepan, combine old-fashioned oats and unsweetened almond milk.

2. Bring to a simmer and cook for about 5-7 minutes, stirring occasionally, until the oats are tender.

3. Stir in sliced ripe banana and ground cinnamon.

4. Drizzle with honey if desired.

5. Enjoy this comforting Cinnamon and Banana Oatmeal.

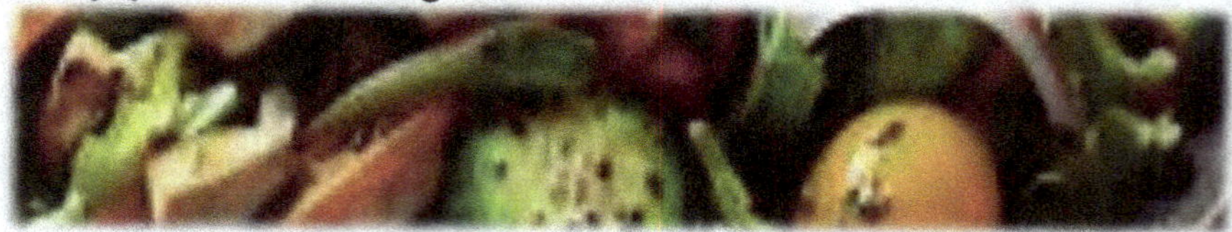

Baked Apples with Cinnamon and Walnuts

Prep Time: 10 mins │ Cook Time: 30 mins │ Servings:1 │ Cal: 75

Ingredients:

- 1 apple (e.g., Granny Smith), cored and halved

- 1/4 tsp ground cinnamon

- 1 tbsp chopped walnuts

- 1 tsp honey (optional)

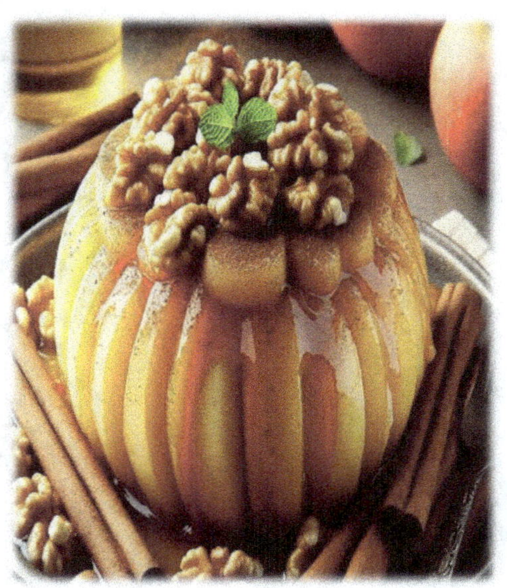

Instructions:

1. Preheat your oven to 350°F (175°C).

2. Place apple halves in a baking dish.

3. Sprinkle with ground cinnamon and top with chopped walnuts.

4. Drizzle with honey if desired.

5. Bake for about 30 minutes until apples are tender.

6. Enjoy these wholesome Baked Apples with Cinnamon and Walnuts.

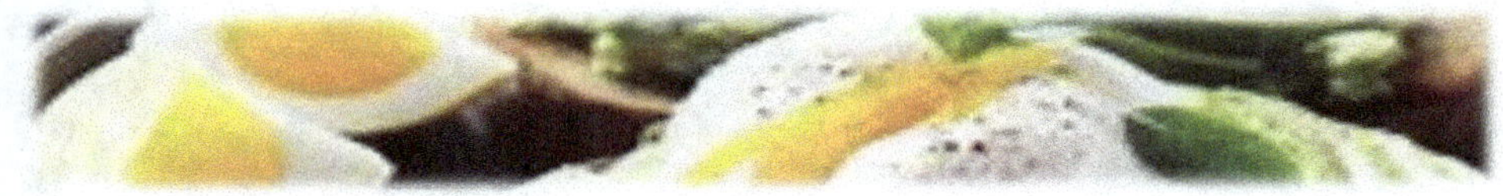

Dark Chocolate-Dipped Strawberries

Prep Time: 10 mins │ Servings: 1 │ Cal: 60

Ingredients:

- 4 ripe strawberries

- 1 oz dark chocolate

(70% cocoa or higher)

- 1 tsp coconut oil

- Chopped nuts

(optional)

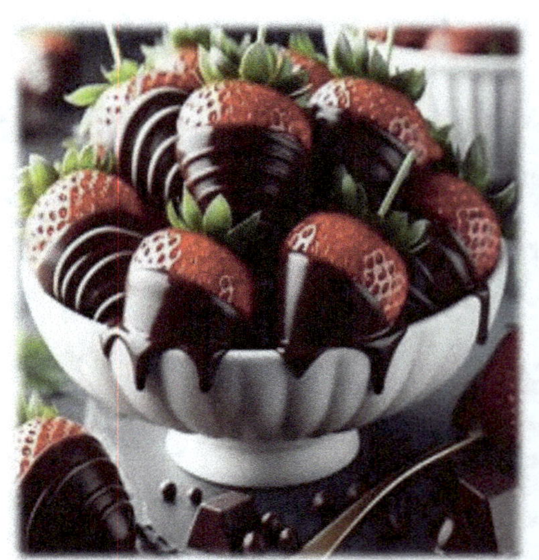

Instructions:

1. Rinse and dry the strawberries thoroughly.

2. In a microwave-safe bowl, melt dark chocolate with coconut oil in 20-second intervals, stirring until smooth.

3. Dip each strawberry into the melted chocolate, allowing the excess to drip off.

4. Place on a parchment-lined tray.

5. Sprinkle with chopped nuts if desired.

6. Let them cool and harden.

7. Enjoy these delightful Dark Chocolate-Dipped Strawberries.

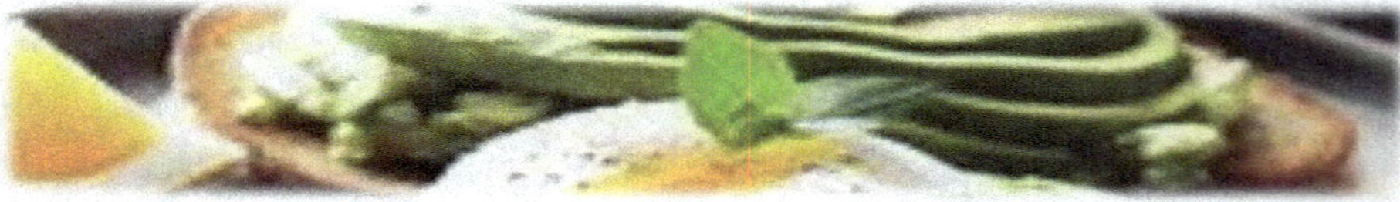

Mixed Berry Parfait with Vanilla Yogurt

Prep Time: 10 mins | Servings:1 | Calories: 250

Ingredients:

- 1 cup mixed berries
(e.g., strawberries,
blueberries, raspberries)
- 1 cup vanilla yogurt
(GERD-safe)
- 2 tbsp granola (optional)
- Fresh mint leaves for
garnish
- Honey for drizzling
(optional)

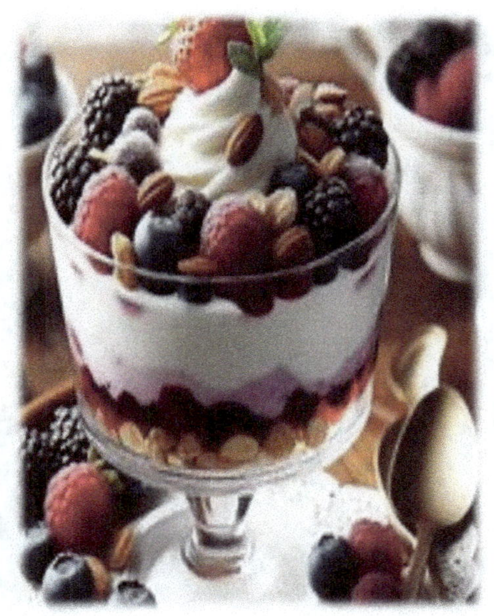

Instructions:

1. In a glass or serving dish, layer mixed berries, vanilla yogurt, and granola (if desired).

2. Garnish with fresh mint leaves.

3. Drizzle with honey if desired.

4. Enjoy this colorful Mixed Berry Parfait with Vanilla Yogurt.

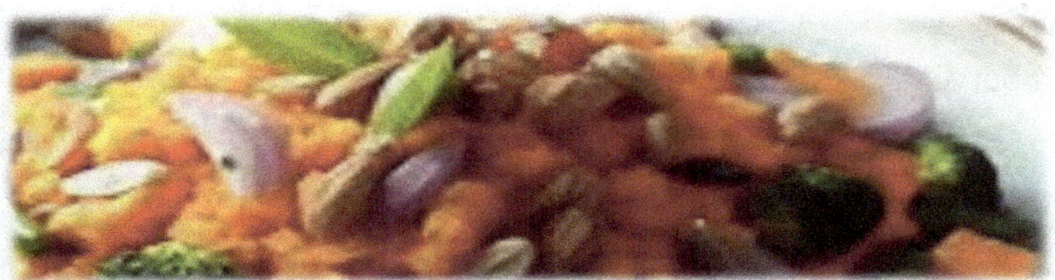

Fruit Salad with Citrus-Mint Dressing

Prep Time: 15 mins │ Servings:1 │ Calories: 75

Ingredients:
- 1/2 cup fresh pineapple chunks
- 1/2 cup fresh mango chunks
- 1/2 cup fresh strawberries, sliced
- 1/2 cup fresh kiwi slices
- Juice of 1/2 orange
- Juice of 1/2 lime
- 1 tbsp fresh mint leaves, chopped
- 1/2 tsp honey (optional)

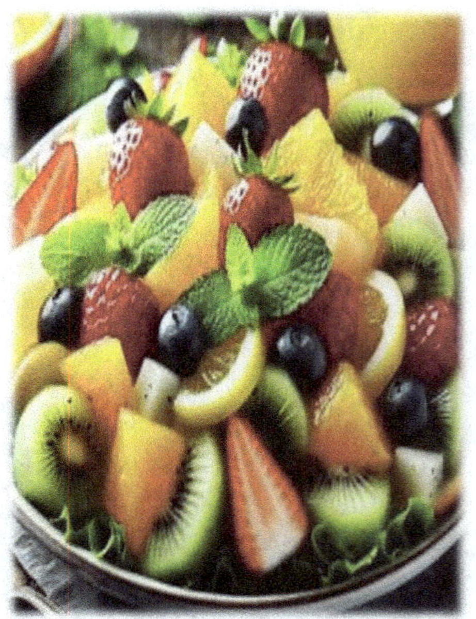

Instructions:

1. In a bowl, combine pineapple chunks, mango chunks, sliced strawberries, and kiwi slices.

2. In a separate bowl, whisk together the orange juice, lime juice, chopped fresh mint, and honey (if desired).

3. Drizzle the citrus-mint dressing over the fruit salad and gently toss.

4. Serve this zesty Fruit Salad with Citrus-Mint Dressing.

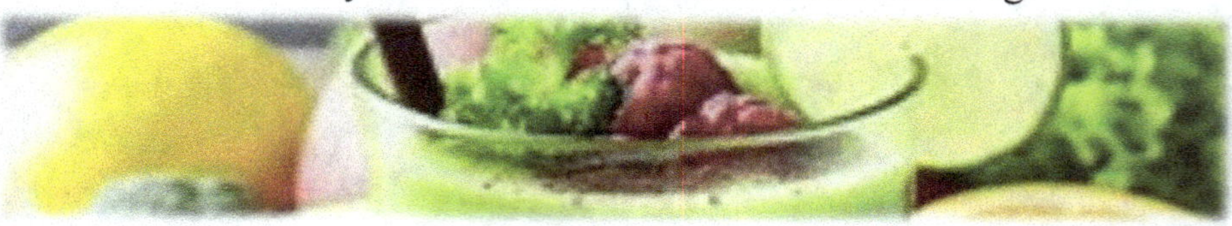

Coconut and Banana Ice Cream

Prep Time: 15 mins | Freezing: 3 to 4 Hrs | Servings:1 | Cal: 73

Ingredients:

- 1 ripe bananas, peeled, sliced, and frozen

- 1/4 cup unsweetened coconut milk

- 1/4 tsp vanilla extract

- Shredded coconut for garnish (optional)

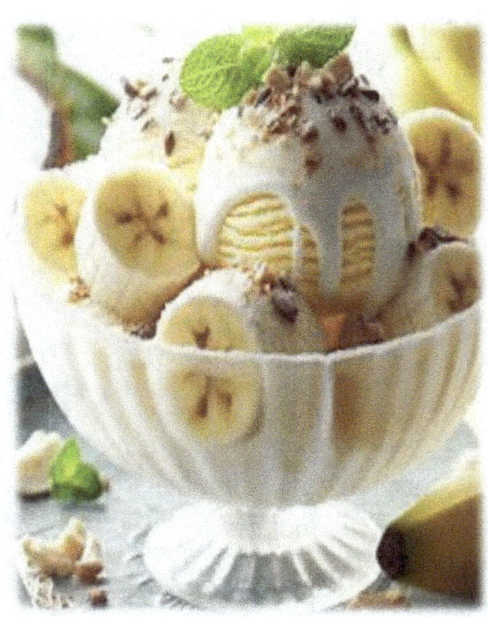

Instructions:

1. In a food processor, blend the frozen banana slices until smooth.

2. Add unsweetened coconut milk and vanilla extract. Blend until well combined.

3. Transfer the mixture to a container and freeze for 3-4 hours.

4. Scoop and serve with shredded coconut if desired.

5. Enjoy this guilt-free Coconut and Banana Ice Cream.

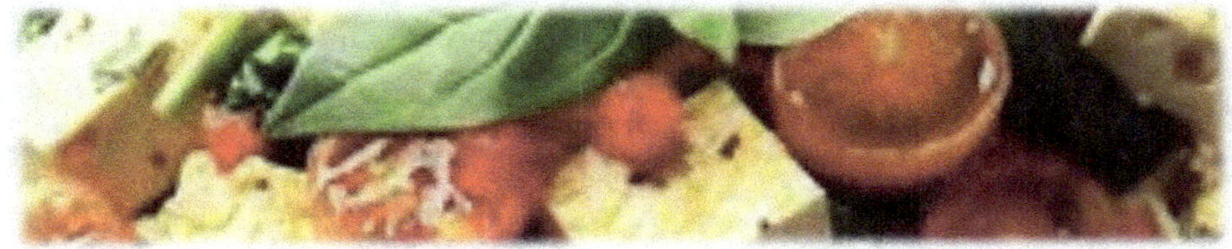

Peach and Blueberry Crisp

Prep Time: 10 mins | Cook Time: 20 mins | Servings:1 | Cal: 150

Ingredients:
- 1 peaches, peeled, pitted, and sliced
- 1/2 cup fresh blueberries
- 1/2 tbsp honey
- 1/4 tsp ground cinnamon
- 1/4 cup old-fashioned oats
- 1 tbsp almond flour
- 1 tbsp chopped almonds
- 1 tbsp coconut oil, melted
- 1/4 tsp vanilla extract

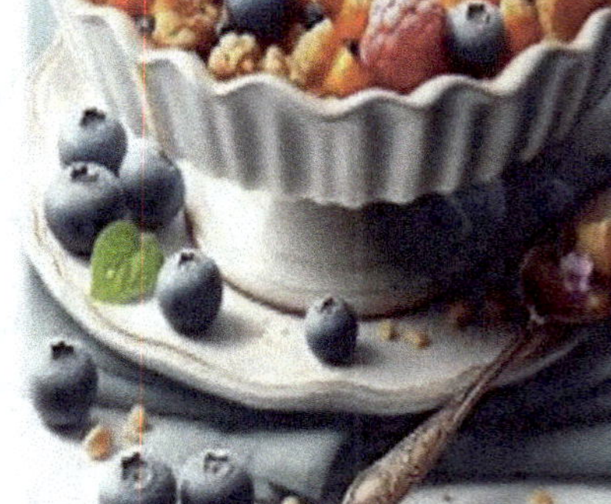

Instructions:
1. Preheat your oven to 350°F (175°C).
2. In a mixing bowl, combine sliced peaches, blueberries, honey, and ground cinnamon. Mix well.
3. In a separate bowl, combine old-fashioned oats, almond flour, chopped almonds, melted coconut oil, and vanilla extract. Mix until crumbly.
4. In individual ramekins or a baking dish, layer the fruit mixture and top with the oat crumble.
5. Bake for about 30 minutes until the top is golden and the fruit is bubbling.
6. Serve this warm Peach and Blueberry Crisp.

Pineapple Sorbet

Prep Time: 10 mins | Freezing: 4 hrs | Servings: 1 | Cal: 50

Ingredients:

- 1 cup fresh pineapple chunks

- 1/4 cup coconut water

- 1/2 tsp honey (optional)

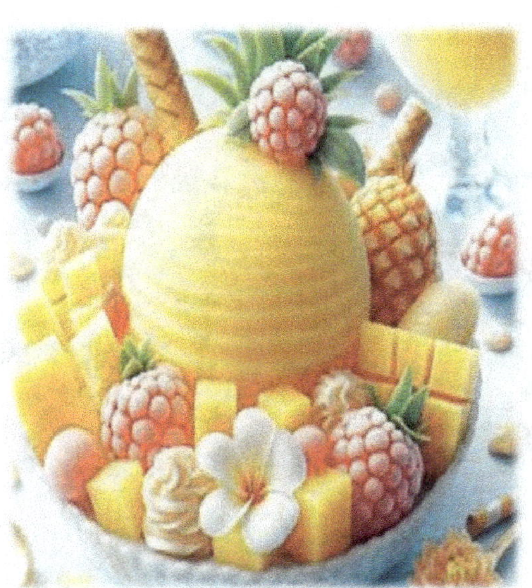

Instructions:

1. In a blender, combine fresh pineapple chunks, coconut water, and honey (if desired).

2. Blend until smooth.

3. Transfer the mixture to a container and freeze for at least 4 hours.

4. Scoop and enjoy this refreshing Pineapple Sorbet.

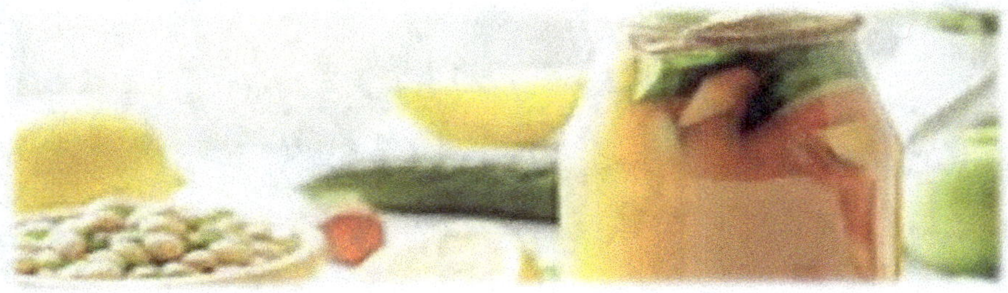

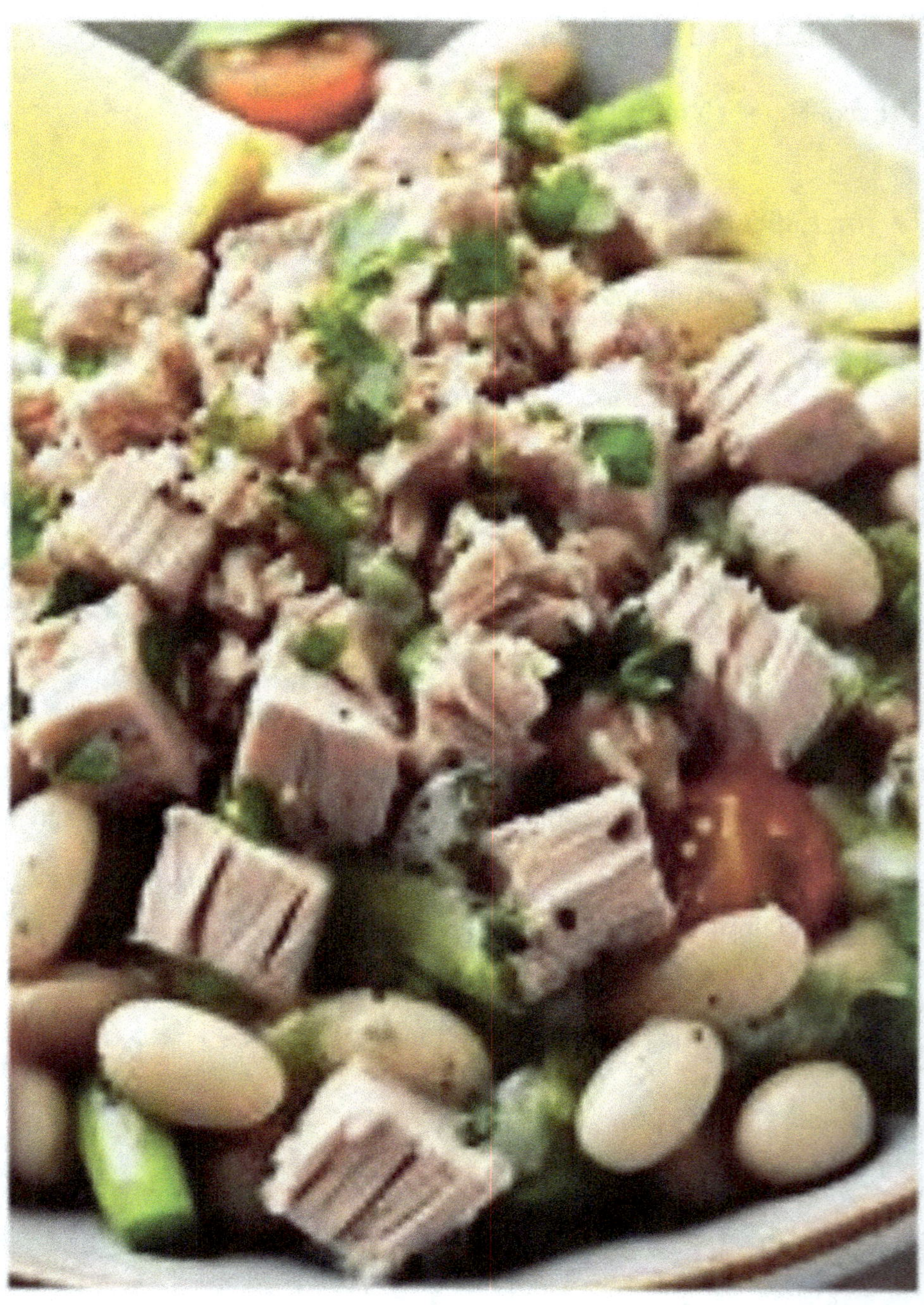

HYDRATING BEVERAGE AND SMOOTHIE RECIPES

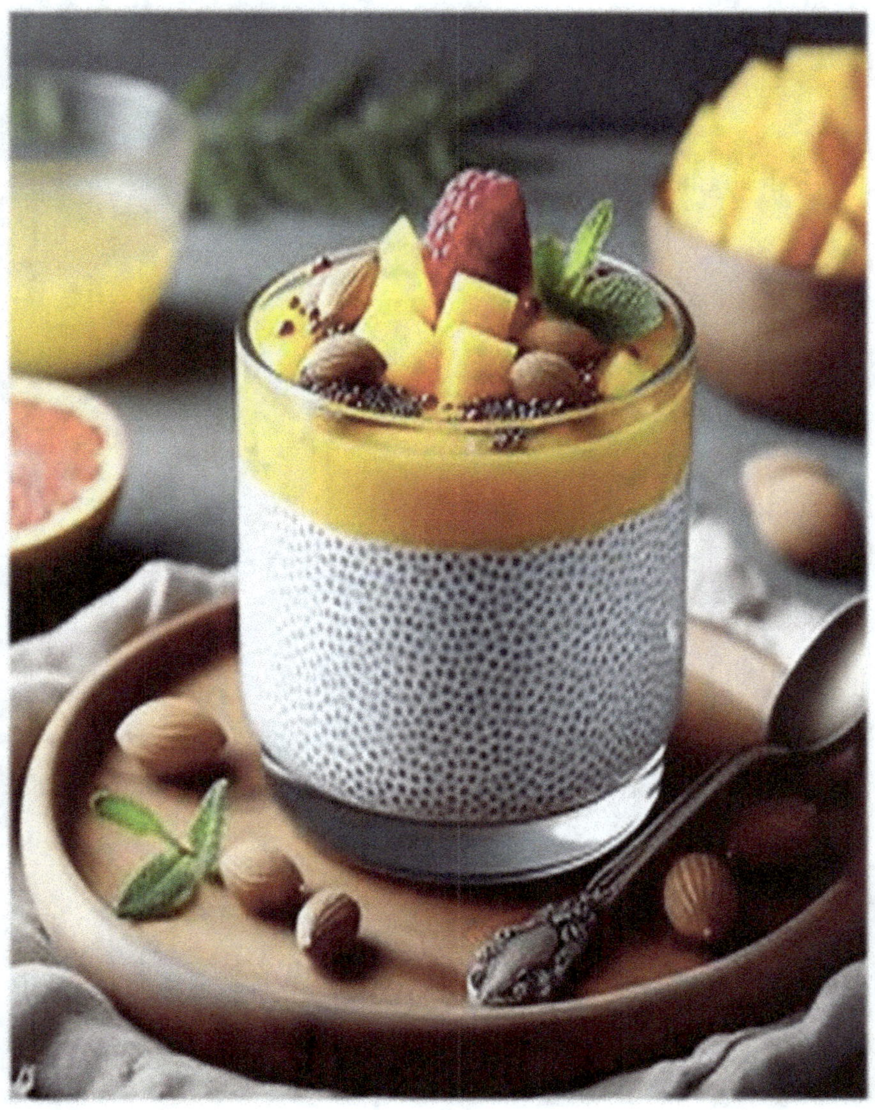

Cucumber and Mint Infused Water

Prep Time: 5 mins | Servings: 1 | Calories: 10

Ingredients:

- 1/2 cucumber, sliced

- 6-8 fresh mint leaves

- 4 cups water

- Ice cubes (optional)

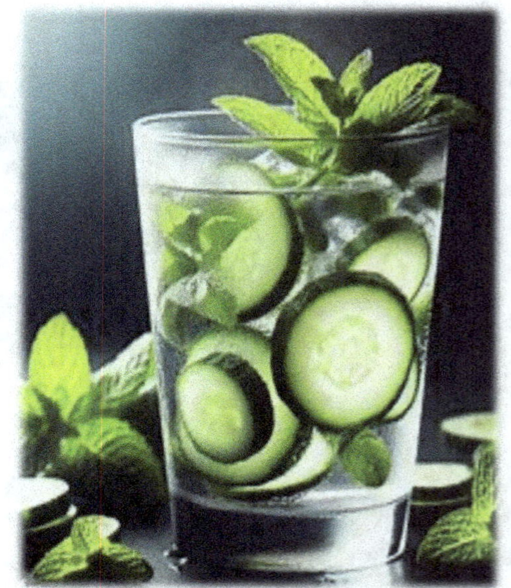

Instructions:

1. Place cucumber slices and fresh mint leaves in a pitcher.

2. Pour in water and add ice cubes if desired.

3. Let it chill in the refrigerator for at least 2 hours to infuse the flavors.

4. Serve and stay refreshed with this Cucumber and Mint Infused Water.

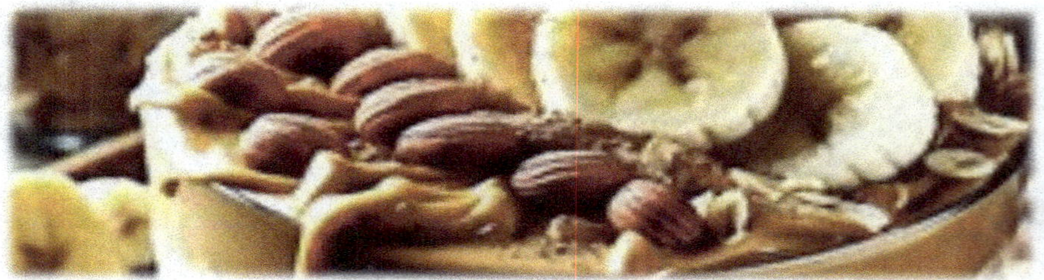

Watermelon and Basil Cooler

Prep Time: 10 mins | Servings: 1 | Calories: 90

Ingredients:

- 2 cups fresh watermelon, cubed

- 4-6 fresh basil leaves

- 1/2 lime, juiced

- 1 cup water

- Ice cubes

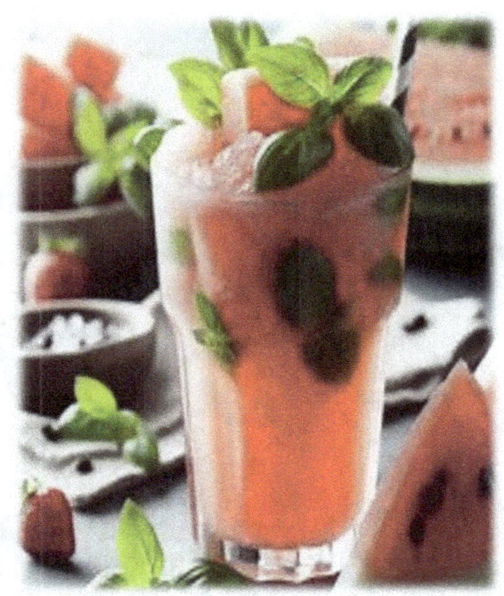

Instructions:

1. Blend fresh watermelon, fresh basil leaves, lime juice, and water until smooth.

2. Add ice cubes to a glass and pour the watermelon mixture over them.

3. Stir gently and savor the Watermelon and Basil Cooler's delightful flavors.

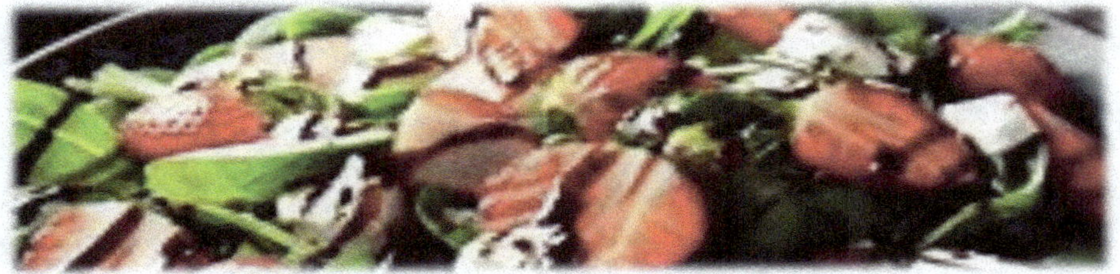

Ginger and Lemon Iced Tea

Prep Time: 10 mins │ Cook Time: 7 min │ Servings: 1 │ Cal: 20

Ingredients:

- 1 cups water

- 1 black tea bag (caffeine-free for GERD)

- 1/2-inch piece of ginger, sliced

- 1 tbsp honey (adjust to taste)

- Juice of 1/2 lemon

- Ice cubes

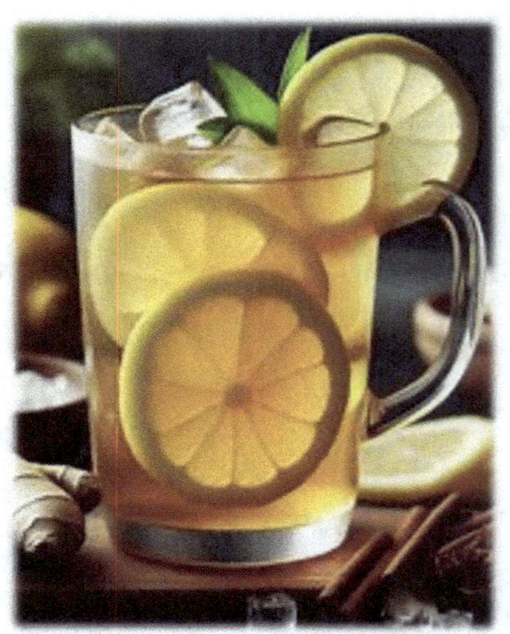

Instructions:

1. In a pot, bring water to a boil. Add tea bags and ginger slices, and steep for about 5 minutes.

2. Remove the tea bags and let the tea cool to room temperature.

3. Stir in honey and lemon juice. Adjust honey to your preferred sweetness.

4. Refrigerate until chilled.

5. Serve with ice cubes for a refreshing Ginger and Lemon Iced Tea.

Pineapple and Coconut Water Refresher

Prep Time: 10 mins │ Servings: 1│Cal: 120

Ingredients:

- 1 cup fresh pineapple

chunks

- 1 cup coconut water

- Ice cubes (optional)

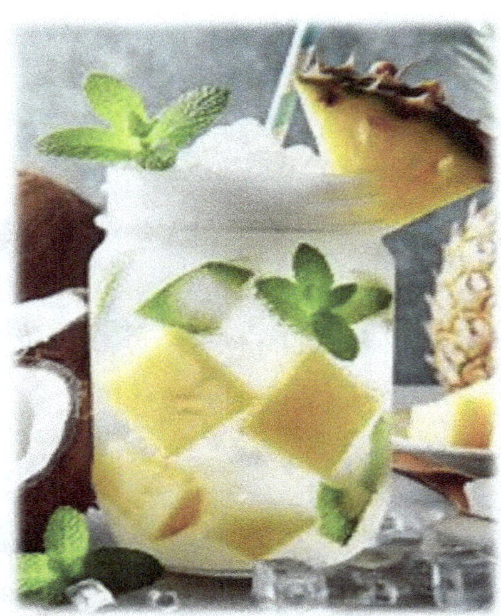

Instructions:

1. Blend fresh pineapple chunks with coconut water until smooth.

2. Add ice cubes to a glass and pour the pineapple-coconut water mixture over them.

3. Enjoy the tropical flavors of the Pineapple and Coconut Water Refresher.

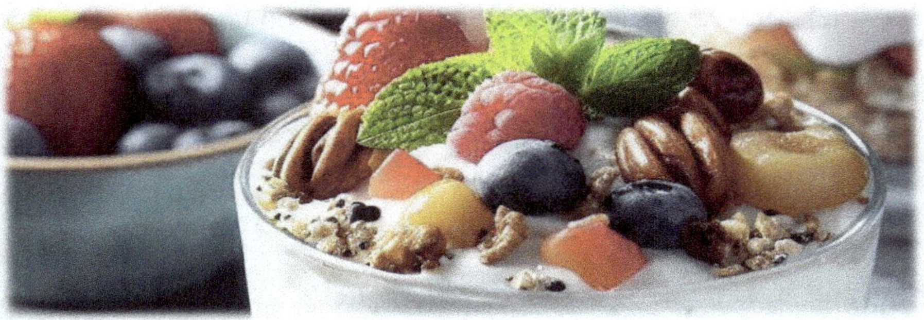

Berry and Green Tea Smoothie

Prep Time: 10 mins | Servings: 1 | Cal: 150

Ingredients:

- 1 cup mixed berries (e.g., strawberries, blueberries, raspberries)
- 1 cup brewed and cooled green tea (caffeine-free for GERD)
- 1/2 banana
- 2 tbsp plain Greek yogurt
- 1 tbsp honey (adjust to taste)
- Ice cubes

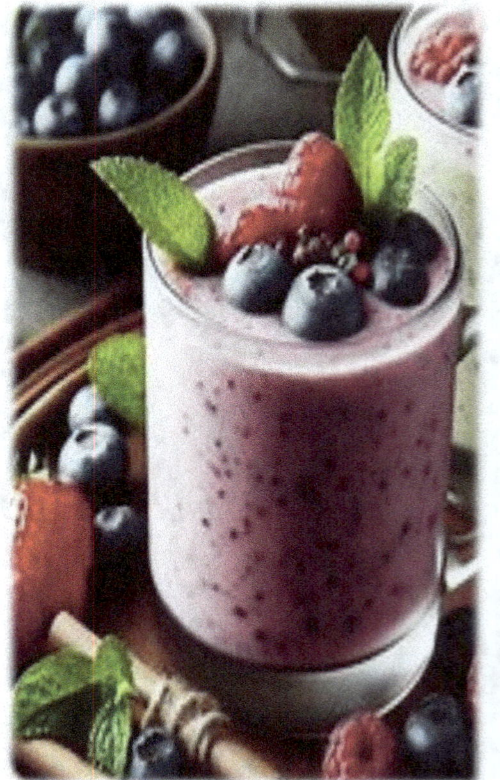

Instructions:

1. Blend mixed berries, green tea, banana, plain Greek yogurt, and honey until smooth.

2. Add ice cubes and blend again for a refreshing and nutritious Berry and Green Tea Smoothie.

Banana and Oatmeal Smoothie

Prep Time: 10 mins │ Servings: 1 │ Cal: 300

Ingredients:

- 1 ripe banana

- 1/2 cup rolled oats

- 1 cup almond milk (or

any non-citrus, non-dairy

milk)

- 1 tbsp honey (adjust to

taste)

- 1/2 tsp cinnamon

- Ice cubes (optional)

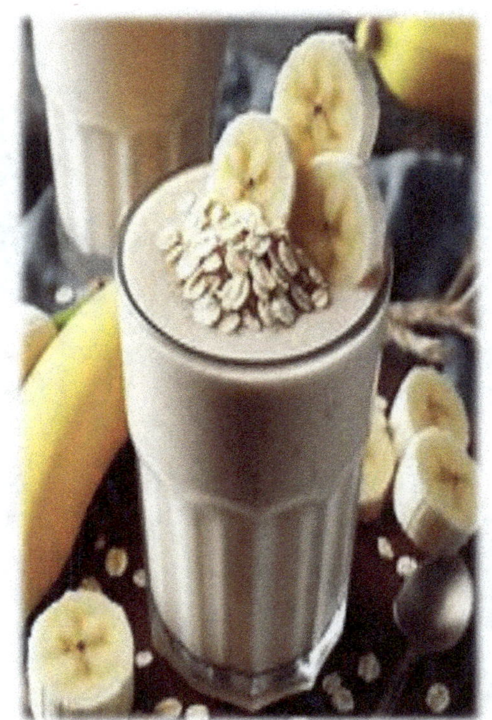

Instructions:

1. In a blender, combine the ripe banana, rolled oats, almond milk, honey, and cinnamon.

2. Blend until smooth.

3. Add ice cubes for extra thickness and blend again.

4. Enjoy the creamy and soothing Banana and Oatmeal Smoothie.

Papaya and Spinach Smoothie

Prep Time: 10 mins | Servings: 1 | Cal: 200

Ingredients:

- 1 cup fresh papaya, cubed
- 1 cup fresh spinach leaves
- 1/2 cup plain Greek yogurt
- 1/2 cup water
- 1 tbsp honey (adjust to taste)
- Ice cubes (optional)

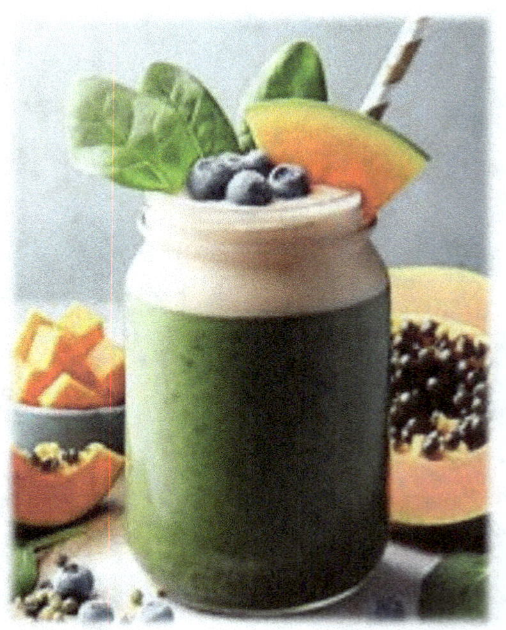

Instructions:

1. Blend fresh papaya, fresh spinach leaves, plain Greek yogurt, water, and honey until smooth.
2. Add ice cubes for extra chill and blend again.
3. Savor the nutrient-packed Papaya and Spinach Smoothie.

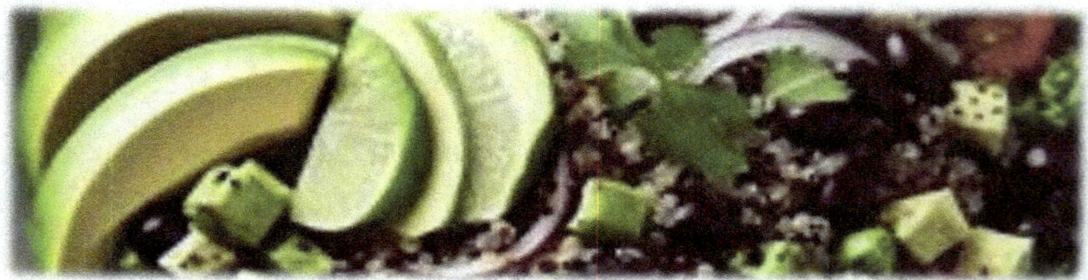

Avocado and Banana Smoothie

Prep Time: 10 mins │ Servings: 1│Cal: 250

Ingredients:

- 1/2 ripe avocado

- 1 ripe banana

- 1/2 cup almond milk
(or any non-citrus, non-
dairy milk)

- 1 tbsp honey (adjust to
taste)

- Ice cubes (optional)

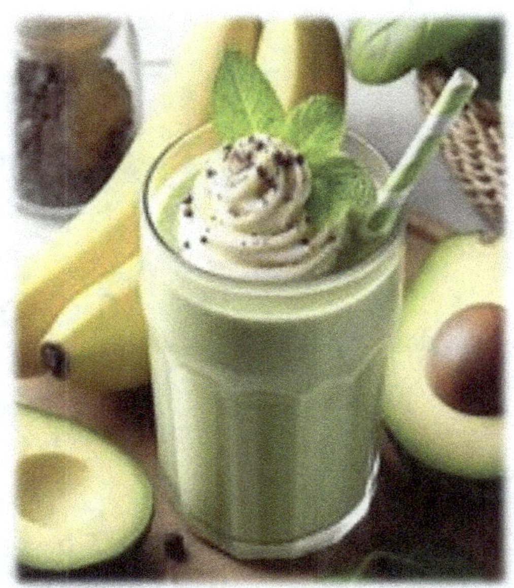

Instructions:

1. In a blender, combine ripe avocado, ripe banana, almond milk, and honey.

2. Blend until creamy and smooth.

3. Add ice cubes for extra chill and blend again.

4. Enjoy the rich and satisfying Avocado and Banana Smoothie.

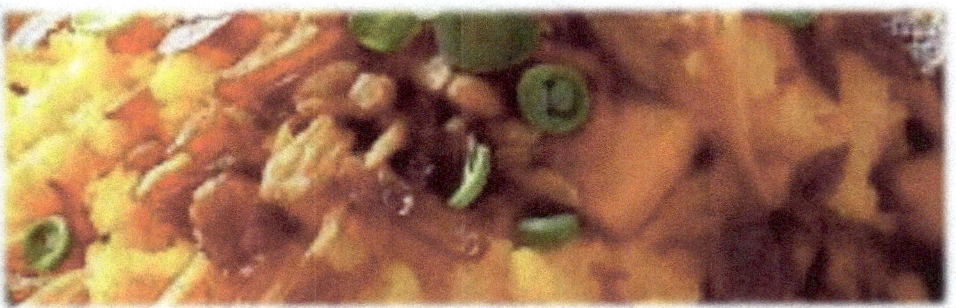

Blueberry and Chia Seed Smoothie

Prep Time: 10 mins │ Servings: 1│Cal: 250

Ingredients:

- 1 cup fresh or frozen blueberries
- 1 cup almond milk (or any non-citrus, non-dairy milk)
- 2 tbsp chia seeds
- 1 tbsp honey (adjust to taste)
- Ice cubes (optional)

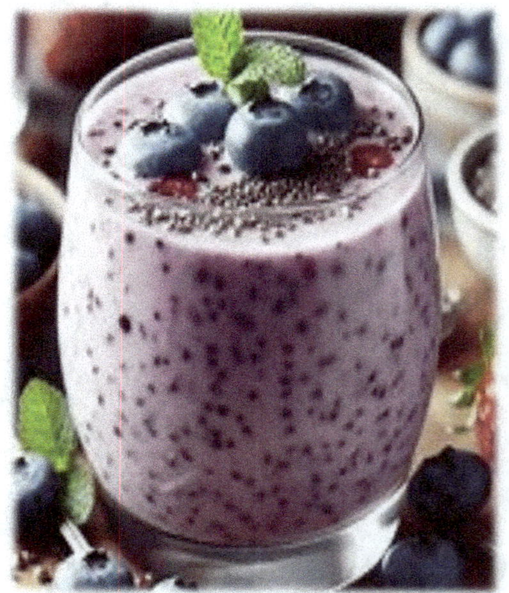

Instructions:

1. In a blender, combine blueberries, almond milk, chia seeds, and honey.

2. Blend until smooth.

3. Add ice cubes for extra thickness and blend again.

4. Enjoy the antioxidant-packed Blueberry and Chia Seed Smoothie.

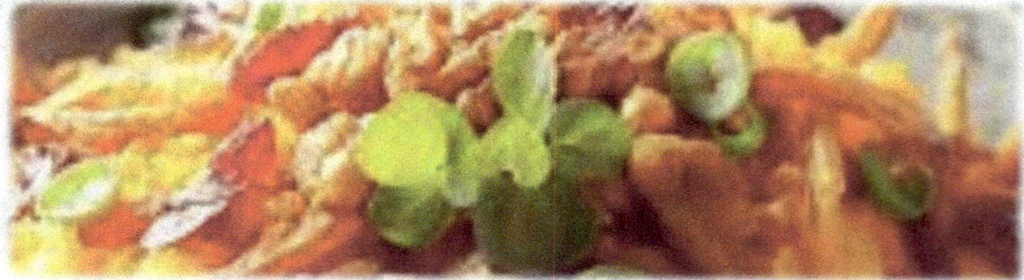

Peach and Almond Smoothie

Prep Time: 10 mins | Servings: 1 | Cal: 300

Ingredients:

- 1 cup fresh or frozen peaches
- 1 cup almond milk (or any non-citrus, non-dairy milk)
- 1/4 cup unsalted almonds
- 1 tbsp honey (adjust to taste)
- Ice cubes (optional)

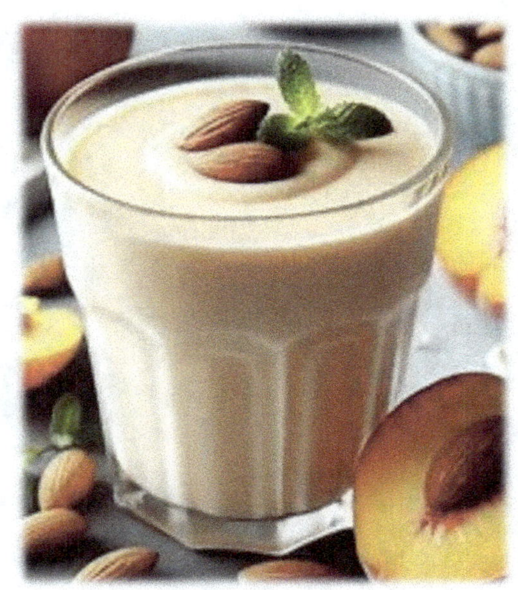

Instructions:

1. In a blender, combine peaches, almond milk, unsalted almonds, and honey.

2. Blend until creamy and smooth.

3. Add ice cubes for extra chill and blend again.

4. Enjoy the delightful Peach and Almond Smoothie.

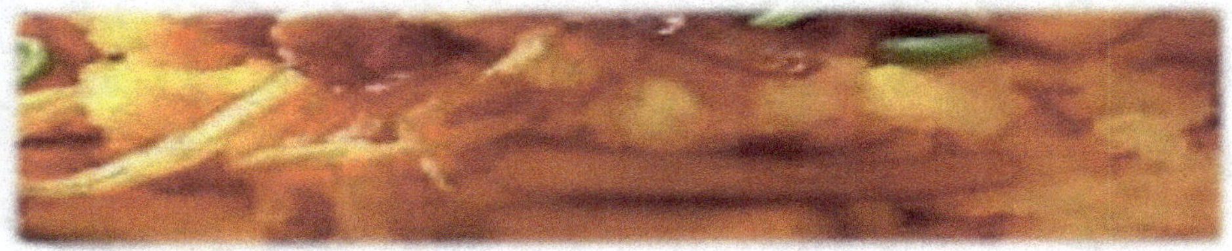

Chamomile and Lavender Tea

Prep Time: 5 mins | Cook Time: 5 mins | Servings: 1 | Cal:0

Ingredients:

- 1 chamomile tea bag

- 1 lavender tea bag

- 2 cups hot water

- Honey (optional, adjust

to taste)

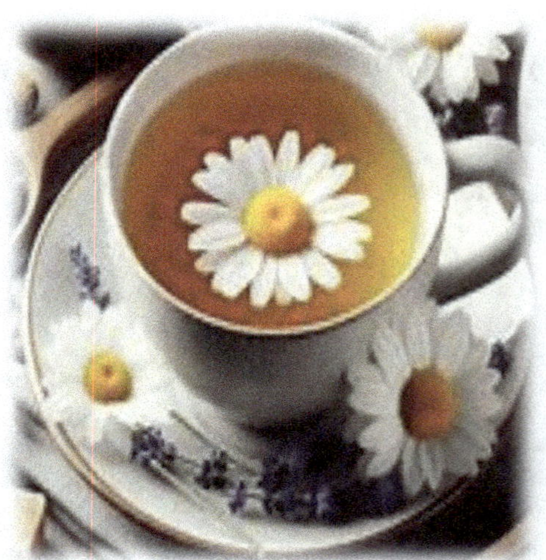

Instructions:

1. Place chamomile and lavender tea bags in a cup.

2. Pour hot water over the tea bags and steep for 3-5 minutes.

3. Remove the tea bags and add honey if desired.

4. Enjoy the gentle and calming Chamomile and Lavender Tea.

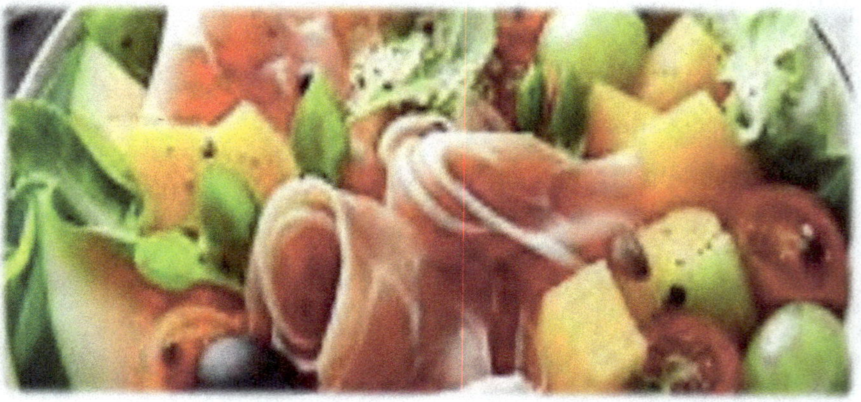

CHAPTER SIX

STRESS MANAGEMENT AND ITS IMPACT ON GERD

Stress is an unwelcome companion in the lives of many, and it has a significant impact on GERD. Let's explore the profound connection between stress and Gastroesophageal Reflux Disease.

- Stress triggers our fight-or-flight response, leading to muscle tension and increased stomach acid production.

- Chronic stress weakens the lower esophageal sphincter, allowing acid to flow back into the esophagus.

Stress-Relief Techniques

- Deep breathing exercises to calm the nervous system.

- Meditation and mindfulness practices.

- Yoga and progressive muscle relaxation.

- Prioritizing sleep to ensure adequate rest.

- Manage time effectively and set realistic goals.

- Seek support through counseling or therapy.

Maintaining a Healthy Weight

Excess weight places additional pressure on the stomach, exacerbating GERD symptoms. Let's delve into the importance of weight management.

- Excess abdominal fat can compress the stomach and promote reflux.

- Weight loss can significantly reduce the frequency and intensity of GERD symptoms.

- Regular exercise to burn calories and improve overall health.

- Develop a balanced, GERD-friendly diet plan.

- Set realistic weight loss goals.

- Eat smaller, more frequent meals to prevent overeating.

- Avoiding late-night snacking to give your stomach time to digest before bedtime.

Exercise and GERD

Exercise is a crucial component of a healthy lifestyle, but it can have a mixed impact on GERD. Let's explore how to strike the right balance

- High-impact, vigorous exercise can increase intra-abdominal pressure, contributing to reflux.

- Gentle, low-impact exercises, like walking and swimming, can help maintain a healthy weight and reduce GERD symptoms.

- Time your workouts to avoid exercising too soon after meals.

- Elevate the head of your bed to prevent nighttime reflux after evening exercise.

- Consulting with a healthcare professional for personalized exercise recommendations.

By addressing these critical aspects of lifestyle, you'll not only manage but potentially alleviate your GERD symptoms. Your well-being is our priority. Is this content satisfactory, or would you like any revisions or additions before we proceed to the next topic?

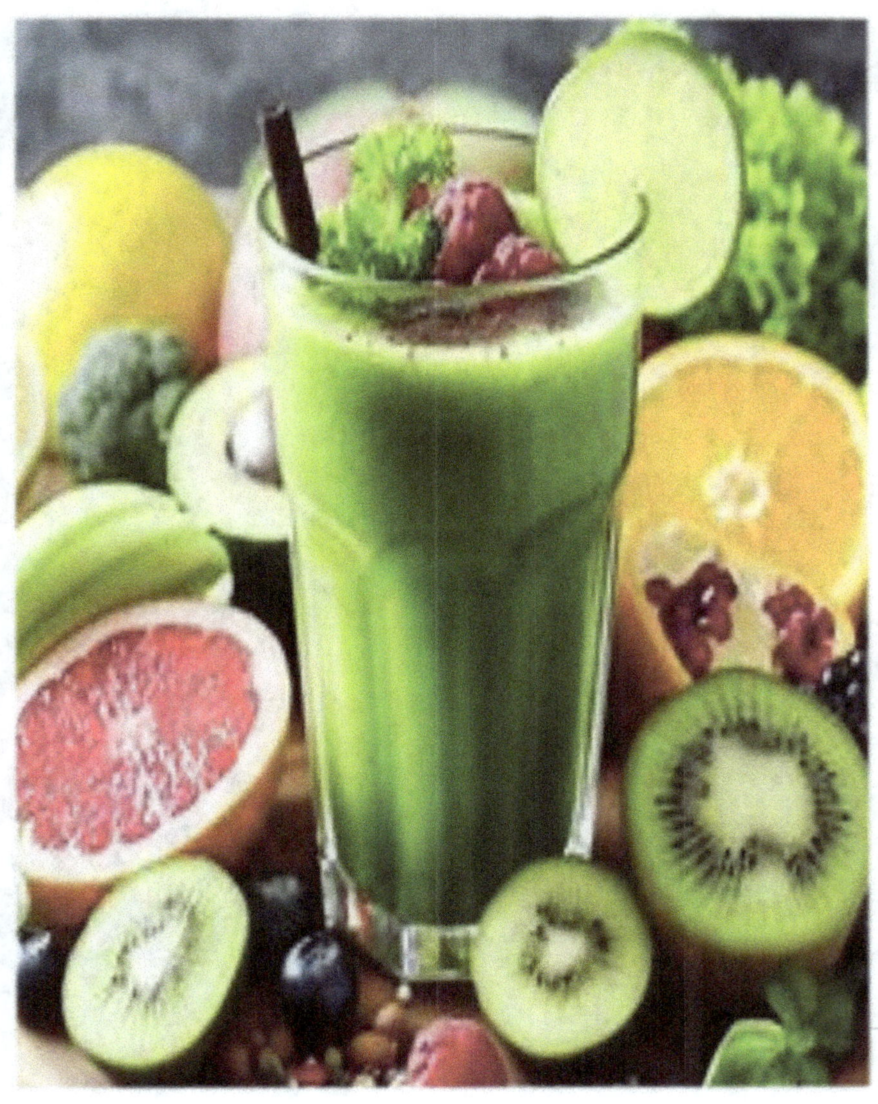

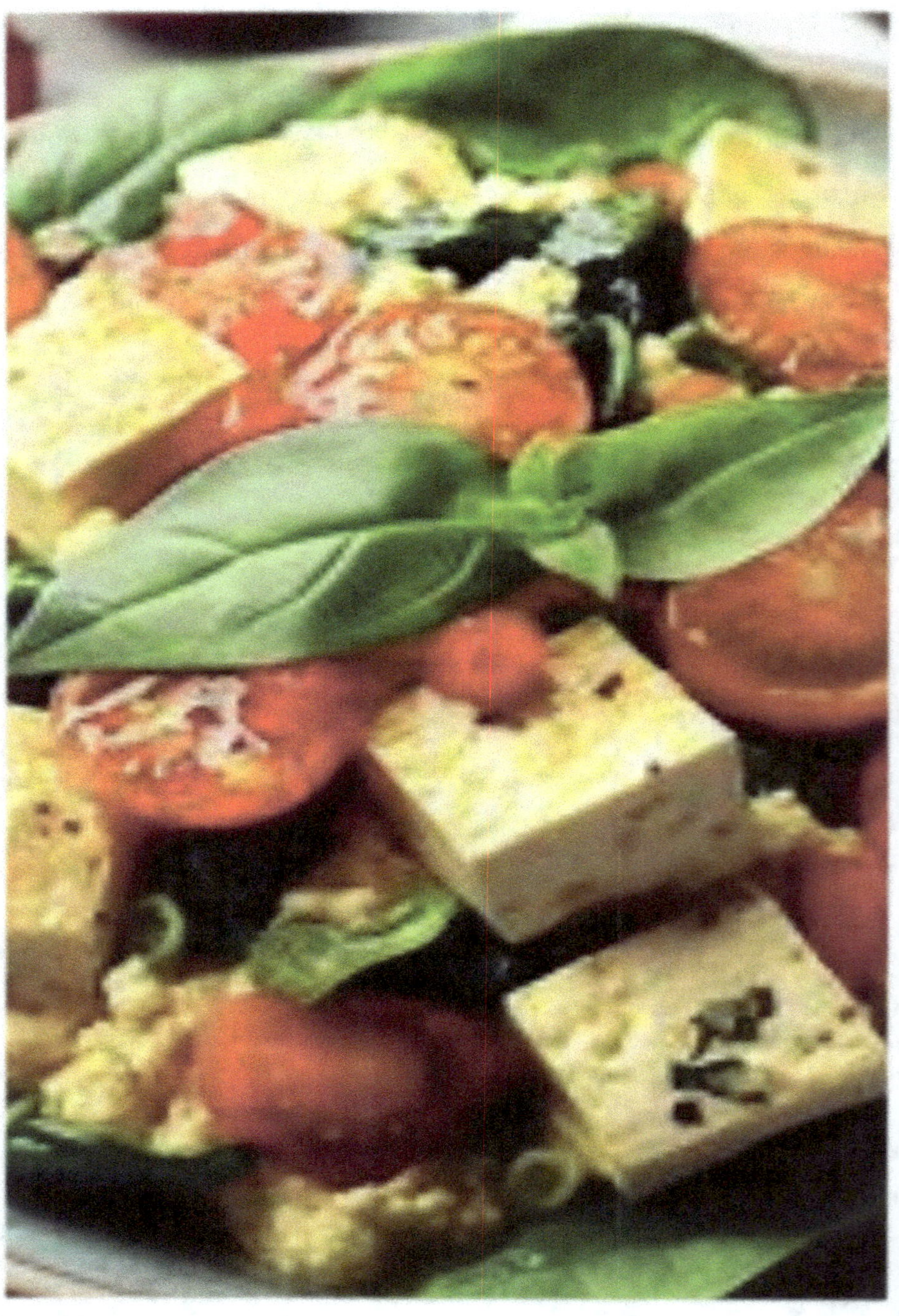

CONCLUSION

As we reach the final pages of this journey, take a moment to reflect on how far you've come. You embarked on this path seeking relief from the relentless grip of Gastroesophageal Reflux Disease, and you've learned that a GERD-friendly diet can be your most powerful ally. The knowledge you've gained, the recipes you've explored, and the changes you've made have all contributed to your journey toward GERD relief.

Remember that healing is not a destination; it's an ongoing journey. Continue to apply the principles you've discovered in this book to keep GERD at bay. Every step you take is a stride toward better health and a life free from the discomfort of heartburn and acid reflux.

Staying committed to a GERD diet may have its challenges, but it's a commitment to your well-being. While you'll undoubtedly face tempting moments and hurdles along the way, know that you have the knowledge, the tools, and the delicious recipes to overcome them. Your commitment is your investment in a life of comfort, health, and vitality.

Don't hesitate to revisit the pages of this book whenever you need guidance and inspiration. The resources and information here are your steadfast companions on this journey.

With your dedication to this newfound lifestyle, you're not merely managing GERD; you're conquering it. The comfort and relief you experience are testaments to the power of your choices.

I'm committed to continuously improving and providing valuable content. Your feedback is invaluable to me. If you've found this book helpful, please share your thoughts, experiences, and any suggestions you may have. Your feedback will help shape future editions and assist others on their journey to GERD relief.

Thank you for joining me on this transformative path toward a healthier, heartburn-free life. Your journey is now a source of inspiration for others, and I hope that your story becomes one of many in a community dedicated to overcoming GERD.

This book is not intended to replace medical advice or treatment. It is meant to complement any medical advice you may have by providing you with information and guidance on how to create a GERD diet plan that works for you. You should always consult your doctor before making any changes to your diet or medication.

With this, we conclude our journey through the "GERD Diet Cookbook for Beginners.

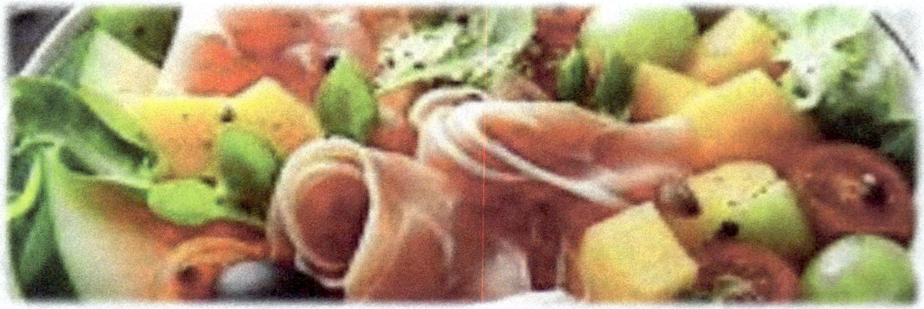

9 798887 164854